Enhancing diagnostics and therapies for rare muscle diseases

Gerry S. Murray

Table of Contents

Chapter 1: The odyssey towards a cure for rare diseases

1.1 Variant interpretation in diagnosis

1.1.1 Challenges in variant interpretation in general

Rare diseases encompass a diverse group of disorders, often characterized by their low prevalence and complex etiology. They affect 3.5% - 5.9% of the worldwide population, of which 72% are genetic [1]. The basis of any kind of treatment is diagnosis. However, the diagnostics of rare genetic diseases present significant challenges in clinical practice. Until recently, the process of obtaining an accurate diagnosis for rare disease patients typically took an average of 4-5 years [2], with many individuals remaining undiagnosed [3,4]. Lack of an accurate diagnosis hinders subsequent treatment development and patients' disease management and family planning [5]. Understanding and addressing the challenges involved in rare disease diagnostics are essential for the advancement of diagnostic practices and the enhancement of patient outcomes.

One challenge in rare disease diagnostics is the substantial clinical variability observed among affected individuals. This variability may partially arise from a polygenic determinism in some rare diseases, where multiple genes contribute to genetic predisposition, and the manifestation of the disease may be influenced by environmental factors [6]. Non-Mendelian inheritance may play a significant role in undiagnosed diseases with unknown etiology [7]. Despite the progress of next-generation sequencing (NGS) [8], challenges persist in deciphering the complex genetic architecture resulting from the complicated interactions and cumulative contributions of multiple genes.

Diagnostics for Mendelian rare diseases pose many challenges as well. While whole-genome sequencing (WGS), facilitated by NGS, has indeed transformed the field of rare disease genomics, its effectiveness in accurately detecting structural variants (SVs) is inherently limited. SVs encompass diverse types of genomic rearrangements such as insertions, deletions, duplications, inversions, and translocations. Short-read sequencing platforms typically produce read lengths of 150-300 base pairs, which poses challenges in capturing large-scale SVs spanning kilobase or megabase ranges. The limitation is evident when dealing with copy number variants (CNVs), such as those found in trinucleotide repeat disorders [9].

With that being introduced, one would naturally assume at least the variant interpretation for single nucleotide variants (SNVs) in Mendelian rare diseases should have been comprehensive, since they are easily detectable by NGS. Unfortunately, this assumption does not hold true. Variant interpretation studies have primarily relied on the analysis of large reference population datasets. The expectation is that by analyzing the depletion of pathogenic variants in the general population, we should be able to identify them effectively. Based on known estimated mutation rates, theoretically, every possible SNV that lacks severe pathogenic effects should exist in at least one living person [10], yet only a small proportion of these variants has been observed in the population. For instance, in the Genome Aggregation Database (gnomAD), which consolidates exome and genome sequencing data from a wide variety of large-scale sequencing projects, only 12% of all possible synonymous variants have been documented [11]. This highlights the need to sequence even larger populations to contribute to a "Comprehensive Variant

Effects Atlas". But for now, human variants remain largely unknown, and even among the small portion that has been known, over half are variants of uncertain significance (VUSs) [12]. This predominance of VUSs stems from the insufficient availability of patient case reports, particularly in rare diseases and the issue was worsened by the ethnic disparity in biomedical databases [13].

It is hoped that an increasing number of newer projects, which prioritize inclusivity, will contribute to addressing these issues. A notable example is the National Institutes of Health (NIH)'s All of Us Research Program, which has set commendable goals for the inclusion of diverse ethnic groups. Currently, over 50% of the enrolled participants are ethnic minorities. With a planned recruitment of 1 million participants, this program holds the potential to significantly improve our understanding of genetic variants [14].

1.1.2 Introduction to deep mutational scanning

Clinical evidence can assist researchers in variant interpretation. Population databases, as aforementioned, as well as variant databases, such as ClinVar and LOVD, allow for the comparison of genetic data from affected individuals with extensive genomic records, facilitating the identification of potential disease-causing variants and associated genes [15]. Large pedigrees of multiple affected families can be constructed using clinical reports to uncover genetic pathology mechanisms [16]. However, these methods have limitations. For example, despite efforts like Matchmaker Exchange to aggregate data from isolated population databases [17,18], rare or ethnically specific variants may still be missing. This could potentially lead to biases in variant interpretation [19]. On the other hand, pedigree segregation analysis could face challenges due to limited case availability and genetic heterogeneity [20].

To complement the insufficient clinical evidence, experimental approaches such as deep mutational scanning (DMS) were developed to unbiasedly generate functional scores for all possible variants [21]. Unlike variant evaluation experiments conducted in animal models, which are undoubtedly valuable but often occur after the variants are identified in patients and can be time-consuming, DMS can equip researchers and clinicians with insights even before specific variants are detected in actual patients. A common DMS workflow consists of two key components: saturation mutagenesis and functional assays to assess variant performance.

Saturation mutagenesis involves introducing all possible variants, such as SNVs or single amino acid substitutions (SAASs), throughout the entire sequence of a specific gene or genomic region [22]. Currently well-established saturation mutagenesis methods include but are not limited to insertion of variant-carrying tiles [23], multiplex homology-directed repair [24] and reversibly-terminated inosine mutagenesis [25]. However, these methods are usually subjected to one or more of the limitations, including intensive labor requirement, high expenses, disparate variant representation, and limited spanning regions. To address these issues, a 2-way extension cloning method called Programmed Allelic Series with Common procedures (PALS-C) was developed and described in this dissertation (2.1.2).

Choosing appropriate functional assays is crucial in obtaining clinically relevant scores that aid in understanding the relationship between variants and disease mechanisms (4.2). Cells rely on well-regulated molecular processes to carry out their functions, and pathological variations can disrupt these processes, leading to disease symptoms. Therefore, the first step in selecting functional assays is to identify the primary disease mechanism. This involves identifying the "disturbance," which refers to the disease-causing variants, and the "consequence," which refers to the cellular phenotypes associated with the disease. In DMS, the disturbance is introduced through saturation mutagenesis, while the consequence is characterized using an appropriate functional assay. The functional assay detects and quantifies specific cellular events resulting from the introduced disturbance. Cytometry-based assays, like fluorescence flow cytometry (FFC), represent the optimal choice for high-throughput analysis in DMS research. These assays often utilize bioreceptors to evaluate cells carrying different variants (4.2.1).

By integrating saturation mutagenesis with well-chosen functional assays, researchers can gain valuable insights into the effects of genetic variants on disease mechanisms and potentially identify new therapeutic targets for intervention. A DMS workflow called Saturation Mutagenesis-Reinforced Functional assays (SMuRF) (Chapter 2).

1.2 Treatment development

1.2.1 Challenges in treatment development for rare diseases in general

Obtaining a definitive diagnosis is merely the beginning of the rest of the long journey towards an effective cure for rare diseases. Until recently, over 90% of rare diseases still lack effective treatments [26]. Developing treatments for rare diseases faces several challenges.

Fundamental challenges include the incomplete understanding of genotype-phenotype relationships and natural history, which hinders trial endpoint development [27,28]. Collaboration among regulatory authorities, researchers, caregivers, and patients is crucial for utilizing natural history data to accelerate the understanding of rare diseases and promote treatment development. Standardized data collection and quantitative model-based data analysis are also prospected to be beneficial in addressing this challenge. Another fundamental challenge is the limited availability of sensitive, non-invasive biomarkers and outcome measures to monitor treatment responses for many diseases [29]. Non-invasive biomarkers are particularly important for patients with muscular diseases, as invasive biopsy procedures can further damage already compromised muscle tissues and have become less desirable due to practical and ethical considerations [30,31].

Another significant challenge in a different aspect is the limitations posed by the common industrial trajectory for treatment development, which is often inapplicable for rare diseases, due to economic considerations concerning the lengthy research and development (R&D) time required and relatively small market sizes [32]. Even when pharmaceutical companies conduct clinical trials for certain rare diseases, strict selection/exclusion criteria are typically imposed [33]. These criteria often prioritize a specific patient population, which may not fully represent the diverse spectrum of the diseases. While the strict criteria for clinical trials are crucial to ensure validity and safety, they can unintentionally exclude patients who may greatly benefit from experimental treatments [34 35].

Personalized medicine offers a new pathway for treatment development by fostering collaborations among academic groups, medical professionals, regulatory teams, and patients [36]. Through this approach, precise treatments can be rapidly developed, particularly benefiting patients with specific mutations or advanced ages and conditions who may have been excluded from company-led clinical trials. A significant challenge in the development of personalized treatments lies in establishing a robust framework to effectively assess the safety and efficacy of these treatments, particularly in the context of n-of-1 trials in rare genetic diseases. Unlike traditional clinical trials involving a larger patient population, n-of-1 trials focus on a single patient with unique mutation(s), making the conventional multi-phase trial scheme incompatible [37]. The development of individualized treatments through n-of-1 trials necessitates the establishment of a new regulatory and ethical framework [38]. A summary of an established trajectory for n-of-1 gene therapy development is described in this dissertation (3.7).

Personalized gene therapies (1.2.2), as well as cell therapies, hold great potential in facilitating the rapid development of precise treatments for patients with rare diseases. It is hoped that these therapies can ultimately achieve a level of accessibility comparable to that of regular prescription medicines. Cell therapy uses living cells, often gene-edited cells derived from the patients themselves, as a drug to treat diseases. A recent notable example is the *ex vivo* cell therapy, exagamglogene autotemcel (exa-cel), developed by

Vertex and CRISPR Therapeutics, for the treatment of sickle cell disease (SCD) and beta-thalassemia. exa-cel involves a bone marrow transplantation using the patient's own, modified cells and is currently seeking approval from the U.S. Food and Drug Administration (FDA) [39].

1.2.2 Challenges and opportunities in gene therapy

1.2.2.1 Gene therapy

Gene therapy involves introducing genetic materials, such as DNA or RNA, into cells to address the root cause of a specific genetic disease, aiming to alleviate or treat the condition. It encompasses gene replacement, gene editing, and gene expression regulation therapies, and has emerged as a promising approach in the field of medicine [40]. Gene therapy holds great promise particularly for rare genetic diseases, offering targeted treatments to counter the underlying genetic mutations [41].

1.2.2.2 Challenges in gene therapy delivery

A significant challenge in gene therapy lies in the delivery process [42]. Specifically in the context of muscle diseases, achieving muscle-specific targeting through a systematic delivery method is of great importance [43]. Non-specific delivery results in the need for higher dosages to achieve expected effects in the target tissue, consequently imposing greater burdens on the patient.

Adeno-associated virus (AAV) is a widely used delivery method for vector-based gene therapies [44]. It is preferred due to its non-integrating nature and lack of association with any human disease [45,46]. However, due to the tendency of AAV particles to accumulate in the liver, non-specific delivery and vector expression can result in hepatotoxicity [47]. Choosing the tissue-specific AAV serotypes and use the tissue-specific expression system can help increase the delivery specificity.

AAV immunogenicity is a major concern [48], as immune responses to AAV particles, including innate, complement, and adaptive immune responses, can have a significant impact on the efficacy and safety of AAV gene therapies. AAV can only be administered once to patients who do not have pre-existing antibodies exceeding a certain threshold [49]. Once a patient develops such antibodies, they can neutralize the AAV particles and render them ineffective for subsequent treatments [50]. Research aiming to engineer adeno-associated virus (AAV) is ongoing, with the goal of evading immune responses and enabling treatment in seropositive patients, as well as facilitating re-administration in previously injected individuals [51,52]. Immune responses to AAV in gene therapy can result in severe associated adverse events. This is especially relevant in the case of muscle diseases, as achieving efficient delivery to muscle tissue and ensuring effective treatment often necessitate high doses of AAV. Furthermore, the adverse events can be exacerbated by advanced disease conditions. This dissertation (3.5) describes a case of an advanced Duchenne muscular dystrophy (DMD) patient who received high-dose AAV gene therapy: the patient exhibited an innate immune response characterized by capillary leak, which tragically resulted in the unexpected death of the patient.

Last but not least, AAV has a restricted capacity, with a maximum genome size of ~5 kb [53,54]. This limitation impacts the design of gene therapy constructs that depend on

AAV delivery (3.3.2). Current solutions to this limitation in the field include designing more compact constructs or incorporating units that can self-assemble [55-57].

Efficiency is another crucial consideration in gene therapy delivery. Antisense oligonucleotides (ASOs) are short synthetic nucleic acid analogs that bind to RNA targets via base pairing, with the aim of reducing gene expression or modifying RNA processing. ASOs, including 2′-O-methoxyethyl (MOE) and phosphorodiamidate morpholino oligomers (PMOs) [58], have been employed in gene expression regulation therapies [59]. However, their delivery efficiency to skeletal muscles and the cardiac muscle is suboptimal [60,61]. To enhance delivery efficiency, modifications, such as cell-penetrating peptide conjugation to ASOs, are currently being developed [62].

1.2.2.3 Diverse gene therapy strategies

1.2.2.3.1 Gene replacement therapy

Gene replacement therapy involves vector-driven delivery of functional genes into the cells to replace defective or non-functional genes. These therapies are primarily aimed at addressing Loss-of-Function (LoF) variants. LoF variants encompass various types, such as nonsense variants that result in premature stop codons, splice site variants that impact protein splicing, frameshift variants caused by insertions or deletions, and loss of the start codon, which impacts gene translation. Additionally, LoF variants also include missense variants that affect protein functions.

The challenges in gene replacement therapy encompass the immunogenicity of the introduced genetic material and/or the corresponding protein product. Since these components are absent in the patients' cells, they can be targeted by the patients' immune system, potentially compromising the safety and efficacy of the therapy [63]. Loss of efficacy over time is another significant challenge in AAV-mediated gene replacement therapy. This can likely be attributed to the gradual reduction of AAV copies [64], and the activation of Toll-like receptor 9 (TLR9)-dependent innate immune responses stimulated by high CpG content, a pathogen-associated molecular pattern (PAMP), present in the viral genome [65,66].

The first AAV-mediated gene therapy approved in the U.S., LUXTURNA developed by Spark Therapeutics, falls under the gene replacement category, which employs *RPE65* gene replacement to treat inherited retinal diseases (IRDs) in patients with *RPE65* mutations [67,68]. Notably, the delivery was accomplished through the use of AAV2 vectors for subretinal injection [69], with limited systemic adverse events observed [70].

Another notable example of gene replacement therapy is ELEVIDYS, developed by Sarepta Therapeutics and recently conditionally approved by FDA [71]. ELEVIDYS will be the first gene therapy for DMD available on the market. While this therapy holds promise [72], there are potential concerns regarding its safety and long-term efficacy [73]. However, currently, there is a lack of sufficient trial data made accessible to researchers in the field.

1.2.2.3.2 Gene editing therapy

Gene editing therapy, on the other hand, employs precise molecular tools, such as transcription activator-like effector nucleases (TALEN) or clustered regularly interspaced short palindromic repeats (CRISPR)-based technologies, to modify specific genomic sites. These tools can be employed to directly correct mutations or introduce desired changes, such as the introduction of exon skipping.

TALENs are engineered restriction enzymes capable of precisely targeting and cutting specific DNA sequences. They are created by fusing a transcription activator-like effector (TALE) DNA-binding domain with a nuclease domain, which possesses the ability to cut DNA strands. TALEs can be engineered to bind to practically any desired DNA sequence, thus making TALEN a versatile gene editing tool [74].

CRISPR systems are components of prokaryotic adaptive immunity that can induce a double-stranded break (DSB) in a specific genomic region guided by a complementary guide RNA (gRNA) sequence [75]. The engineered CRISPR-Cas9 system, widely utilized for gene knockout applications, functions by initiating error-prone DNA repair mechanisms at the targeted DSB. The repair can lead to random insertions or deletions (indels), resulting in frameshift mutations that effectively knock out the targeted gene [76]. Indels introduced near splicing sites have the capability to induce exon skipping, which offers the potential to exclude exons carrying mutations. Exon skipping can restore the protein's reading frame, leading to the generation of a truncated protein that retains a significant degree of functionality. The application of this approach is currently being extensively pursued in the context of DMD mutations [77,78]. Additionally, the combined usage of two gRNAs to create two DSBs on the chromosome enables the targeted deletion of a specific genomic region [79,80]. This strategy was utilized in the first clinical trial that delivered CRISPR constructs into the human body for gene therapy

(EDIT-101 by Editas Medicine and Allergan), which was aimed at restoring vision loss in Leber congenital amaurosis type 10 (LCA10) [81,82]. The application of the dual-gRNA strategy has also been explored for the purpose of deleting *DMD* exons that harbor mutations [83].

One major concern associated with nuclease-based gene editing therapies is the potential occurrence of off-target editing [84]. This concern becomes particularly alarming when there is a risk of unintentionally disrupting cancer suppressor genes. Furthermore, in AAV-mediated gene editing experiments, the observation of viral genome integration at the editing site raises significant concerns [85]. These concerns can be partially addressed through improved design [86], and comprehensive evaluation in pre-clinical experiments [87,88]. Another approach is to develop and utilize DSB-independent editing tools, such as the base editors. Base editors are a class of gene editing tools that enable precise changes to individual nucleotides [89]. Instead of utilizing fully catalytically active Cas proteins, they rely on engineered Cas proteins, such as Cas nickase, which can only induce a single-stranded break, or dead Cas (dCas) proteins, which lack cleavage activity entirely. Well-established base editors comprise the cytosine base editor (CBE), which enables the substitution of C to T [90], and the adenine base editor (ABE), which enables the substitution of A to G [91]. Additional base editors have been developed to expand the existing repertoire, awaiting further validation in their potential therapeutic applications [92-94].

More significantly, the advent of Prime Editing (PE) represents a groundbreaking advancement. By combining a PE protein comprising a Cas nickase domain and a reverse transcriptase (RT) domain with a prime editing guide RNA (pegRNA), PE has the capability to introduce small insertions, small deletions, and all types of point mutations at the targeted site. In principle, this approach could correct up to 89% of known genetic variants associated with human diseases [95]. A significant challenge in utilizing Prime Editing (PE) for clinical trials is its overly large size, rendering it incompatible with AAV-mediated delivery. It is hoped that through further engineering efforts, the size of PE can be reduced to overcome this limitation [96]. Interestingly, I have invested efforts for this aim as a passion project yet failed to generate any promising result (Fig. 1.2.2.3.2.1). Nevertheless, the exploration of using base editors or PE to correct DMD mutations has yielded promising results by others [97,98].

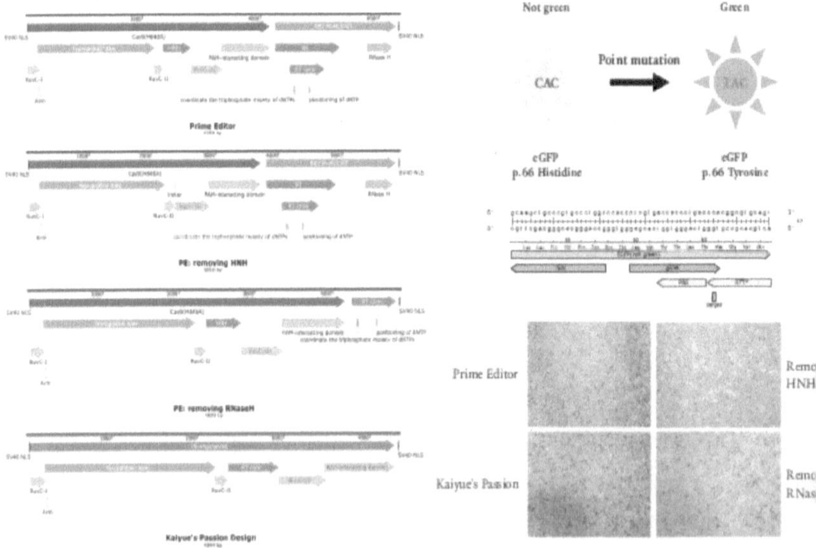

Fig. 1.2.2.3.2.1 Failed engineering effort to reduce the size of the prime editor. Three designs were proposed: (1) removing the HNH domain that is catalytically inactive in PE; (2) removing the RNaseH domain that is in principle not required by PE; (3) "Kaiyue's Passion": removing HNH and inserting the

RT core domain to where HNH was. A stable HAP1 cell line expressing eGFP(Y66H) was established. Prime editing pegRNA and nicking gRNA were design to achieve H to Y editing. eGFP signal serves as a reporter for successful editing. Only the original prime editor resulted in eGFP signal, while cells treated with the other two rational designs and "Kaiyue's Passion" failed to glow. Transfection was performed with Lipofectamine 3000. This experiment was not repeated. PBS: primer binding site; RTT: RT template. Asterisk denotes that the RTT carries the desired mutation in the pegRNA.

1.2.2.3.3 Gene expression regulation therapy

Gene expression regulation therapies aim to enhance or reduce the activity of specific genes, regulating their impact on cellular processes and disease progression.

ASOs have been employed in experiments with the aim of developing gene expression regulation therapies. ASOs can selectively target the start codon of genes, effectively impeding their translation and achieving knockdown. For instance, a peptide-conjugated PMO (PPMO) was used to selectively inhibit the expression of New Delhi metallo-β-lactamase (NDM-1), which enables resistance to carbapenem in bacterial pathogens [99]. ASOs have also been shown to enhance gene translation by selectively targeting the translational inhibitory elements in the 5' untranslated regions (UTRs) of genes [100]. By targeting the 3' end of the coding region, ASOs have the potential to reduce mRNA levels in a translation-dependent, RNase H1-independent manner [101]. In addition, ASOs have been extensively investigated for their potential to target the 3' UTR of *DUX4*, the toxic gene implicated in facioscapulohumeral muscular dystrophy (FSHD) [102-104].

CRISPR-based tools represent another avenue for gene expression regulation therapies, which typically involve the fusion of dCas9 with various effectors to achieve either gene up-regulation or gene down-regulation [105]. While dCas9 does not induce DSBs, the concerns of off-target effects persists [106]. Precautions, such as conducting *in silico* evaluations of off-target effects, should be taken [107]. However, peculiar results have been reported, where bioinformatic approaches failed to reveal predicted off-target sites [108]. This again emphasizes the significance of conducting WGS or targeted sequencing to assess off-target effects when utilizing CRISPR-based tools.

CRISPR interference (CRISPRi) is typically accomplished by fusing dCas9 with a repressor domain such as Krüppel-associated box (KRAB) [109], or other more recent generation systems [110]. On the other hand, CRISPR activation involves the fusion of dCas9 with various transcriptional activators (1.2.3). These tools collectively offer alternative therapeutic approaches to CRISPR gene editing. However, since CRISPRi/a systems also rely on AAV-mediated delivery, they are limited to a one-time-only administration as well. Whether CRISPRi/a exhibits durable effects similar to gene editing [111], or faces the same concerns as gene replacement requires further research [112].

In summary, the development of gene therapy has provided new possibilities for treating previously incurable or challenging diseases. Promising results have emerged from clinical trials. However, further research is necessary to ensure the long-term safety, efficacy, and accessibility of gene therapy.

1.2.3 Introduction to CRISPRa gene therapy

1.2.3.1 Diverse CRISPR activation strategies

The Cas endonuclease activity can be inactivated by point mutations (*e.g.*, D10A and H840A in SpCas9; D832A and E925A in LbCpf1), resulting in a nuclease-deactivated Cas (dCas) incapable of cleaving DNA but still retaining its DNA binding ability [113,114]. In CRISPRa, dCas functions as a homing device to the transcription start sites, and when combined with diverse transcriptional effectors, it can promote gene expression without modifying the genomic sequence [115]. These transcriptional effectors can either facilitate the assembly of the transcription machinery or catalyze epigenetic remodeling at the target sites.

The first-generation CRISPRa platforms utilized dCas9 fused to transcriptional activators such as VP16 or p65 to enhance gene activation [109]. Increasing the number of VP16 activation domains fused to dCas9 resulted in higher gene activation, with VP192 exhibiting the highest activity [116]. VP64, composed of four VP16 domains, is the most commonly used transcriptional activator [117]. The construct employed for the clinical trial described in this dissertation was d*Sa*Cas9-VP64 (3.3.1). A study also demonstrated that fusing two VP64 domains to both the N- and C-terminus of dCas9 improved activation capacity compared to single VP64 fusion [118], yet our *in vivo* mouse study using such a construct detected viral genome rearrangement event (Fig. 1.2.3.1.1 and Fig. 3.3.2.4g-i).

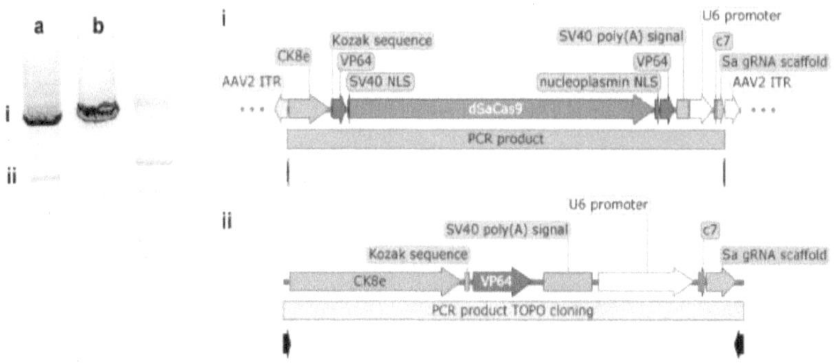

Fig. 1.2.3.1.1 Viral genome rearrangement detected in AAV-injected mice. a, Template DNA was harvested from the liver of an AAV-injected mice. **b,** The dual-VP64 AAV plasmid used to package the virus. **i,** The expected PCR product representing the correct viral genome. **ii,** The truncated viral genome. Sequence was determined using TOPO cloning. Since the *in vivo* efficacy is significantly lower than the *in*

vitro efficacy (3.3.2), we suspected that this detected rearrangement may not be the only rearrangement that occurred.

Second-generation activation CRISPRa platforms, such as synergic activation mediator (SAM), VPR, and SunTag, were developed to achieve more potent and robust gene activation. SAM utilizes dCas9-VP64 with modified sgRNA to recruit additional activation domains (p65 and HSF1) through MS2 hairpins, resulting in a total of twelve activation domains [119]. VPR fuses VP64, p65, and Rta to dCas9, recruiting six activation domains [115]. We also explored VPR for in the pre-clinical experiments described in the dissertation (3.3). The SunTag system uses a repeating peptide array to recruit multiple copies of VP64, achieving a total of 40 activation domains (10 VP64 units) [120]. Although second-generation platforms show increased potency, their larger size requires multiple AAV vectors for *in vivo* delivery, reducing delivery efficiency. Furthermore, the clinical translatability of dual-vector AAV administration is currently lacking, and first-generation platforms may be preferred for achieving desired gene expression levels depending on the gene and application.

Epigenome-modifying enzyme fusion to dCas systems offers an alternative strategy for targeted gene activation by modifying chromatin state. For instance, fusion of dCas9 to p300 or PRDM9 enables histone acetylation or methylation, respectively, resulting in gene activation [121,122]. However, once again, the larger size of these enzymes limits their *in vivo* translatability.

Factors such as gRNA length [123], proximity to the transcription start site (TSS) (typically -400 to -50 bp upstream) [124], and chromatin accessibility [125] influence the effectiveness of CRISPRa platforms. When designing CRISPRa experiments, it is crucial to take these factors into consideration.

Off-target effects in CRISPRa experiments can occur in various scenarios (Fig. 1.2.3.1.2). Primary off-target effects involve nonspecific binding of the dCas9-activator complex to unintended genomic regions, either through guide-dependent or guide-independent mechanisms. Computational prediction methods and chromatin remodeling analysis can help identify primary off-target effects [126]. However, a pitfall of computational prediction is its reliance on the reference human genome, which fails to account for the genetic variations present in the genome of each individual, potentially affecting prediction accuracy [127]. Secondary off-target effects arise from the nonspecific activation of transcriptional networks, resulting in differentially expressed genes. RNA-seq is commonly used to detect secondary off-target effects. Tissue and cell line specificity should also be considered for off-target analysis, especially in *in vivo* studies.

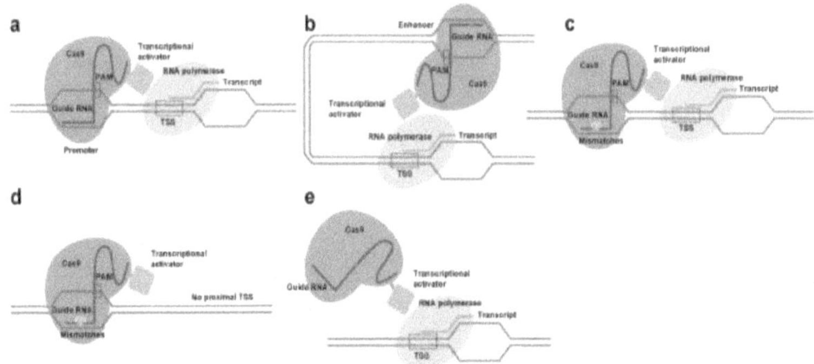

Fig. 1.2.3.1.2 **Example scenarios of on-target and off-target CRISPRa binding.** Example of dCas9-activator complex on-target binding to **a**, promoter region upstream of TSS or **b**, enhancer region upstream of TSS. Example of dCas9-activator complex off-target binding **c**, due to sgRNA mismatch with genomic DNA. Proximity to TSS activates unintended gene, **d**, in intergenic region that does not result in gene

activation, or e, guide-independent activator binding to DNA or DNA/bound proteins that leads to up-regulation of gene expression.

1.2.3.2 Substitute Isoform Rescue (SIR)

Through natural selection, genomes gained redundancy either to expand the genetic versatility or serve as contingency plans to counter genetic mutations. Redundancy can take the form of redundant genes or gene isoforms, and interestingly, they can demonstrate transcriptional responsiveness to the absence of their redundant partners, with their conditional up-regulation serving as a responsive backup circuit [128]. Such genomic redundancy has huge therapeutical potentials when accompanied with rational design [129].

One prominent example of utilizing a redundant gene is the gene therapy approach devised for spinal muscular atrophy (SMA) [130]. Humans possess two Survival Motor Neuron (SMN) genes, *SMN1* and *SMN2*. Loss or mutations of *SMN1* cause SMA, while loss of *SMN2* is generally not associated with the disease [131]. The duplication event of the *SMN* gene occurred during the evolution of non-human primates, with SMN2 being unique to *Homo sapiens* [132]. *SMN1* and *SMN2* differ by only 5 nucleotides, including a critical C-to-T transition in exon 7 of *SMN2*, which, despite being translationally silent, leads to altered splicing patterns resulting in predominantly exon 7-lacking *SMN2* transcripts (~90%) and a smaller fraction of full-length *SMN2* transcripts [133]. SMA patients typically have 2-3 copies of *SMN2*, allowing for partial compensation with approximately 10-30% of full-length SMN protein production [134].

Gene therapies have been developed to capitalize on this redundancy, with available treatments such as Spinraza (ASOs) and Evrysdi (small molecules) aiming to inhibit exon 7 skipping in SMN2 or modulate exon 7 inclusion, respectively. Additionally, multiple *SMN2* gene editing strategies are being developed to either directly inhibit undesired exon 7 skipping or modify the crucial C-to-T transition to match that of *SMN1* [135].

We have proposed an innovative strategy called Substitute Isoform Rescue (SIR) to harness the therapeutic potential of genomic redundancy. Gene isoforms are mRNA variants generated from the same genomic locus, exhibiting differences in TSSs, coding sequences (CDSs), and/or UTRs. These variations have the potential to modulate gene expression patterns and functional outcomes [136,137]. SIR was developed on the principle that if a mutation affects the canonical isoform of a tissue but not another isoform, the unaffected isoform can be up-regulated to compensate for the mutation.

SIR was employed to develop a gene therapy for a DMD patient who had a deletion that eliminated the DNA sequence encoding exon 1 of the dystrophin muscle isoform (3.1 and 3.2). There are three full-length dystrophin isoforms known (muscle, purkinje, cortical), differing only in their promoter and exon 1 sequence to each other [138] (Fig. 1.2.3.2.1).

	1	2	3	4	5	6	7	8	9	10	11	12	13	14	15	16	17	18	19	20
Muscle	M	L	W	W	E	E	V	E	D	C	Y	E	R	E	D	V	Q	K	K	T
Purkinje				M	S	E	V	S	S	D	-	E	R	E	D	V	Q	K	K	T
Cortical									M	E	D	E	R	E	D	V	Q	K	K	T

Fig. 1.2.3.2.1 Amino acid sequence alignment of the N-termini of the full-length dystrophin isoforms. The known full-length dystrophin isoforms differ from one another by only a few amino acids

Up-regulation of non-muscle dystrophin isoforms has been observed in DMD patients that display milder muscle pathology and also in dystrophinopathy patients who manifest in X-Linked Dilated Cardiomyopathy (XLDCM) without an overt skeletal muscle phenotype [139,140]. We therefore hypothesized that up-regulation of full-length non-muscle isoforms of dystrophin can functionally compensate for the absence of muscle dystrophin, and that this can be used as a therapeutic strategy for patients with *DMD* mutations in the promoter, exon 1 and intron 1 of the muscle isoform. Dystrophin cortical isoform up-regulation was successfully achieved using a CRISPRa construct in both *in vitro* and *in vivo* settings, as described in this dissertation (3.3 and 3.4).

2.1 Establishment of Saturation Mutagenesis-Reinforced Functional Assays (SMuRF)

2.1.1 Dystroglycanopathies: Where No SMuRF Had Gone Before

Dystroglycanopathies are a set of rare autosomal recessive diseases with clinical heterogeneity ranging from brain malformation in Walker-Warburg syndrome (WWS) to milder muscular symptoms in Limb-Girdle Muscular Dystrophies (LGMDs) [141]. The most severe dystroglycanopathy cases can lead to miscarriage and neonatal deaths, highlighting the critical need for a better understanding of the clinical significance of variants in genetic testing. [142-144]. Most known dystroglycanopathy cases are caused by missense variants [145]. Pathogenic variants in *DAG1*, the gene that encodes alpha-dystroglycan (α-DG), and genes encoding enzymes involved in α-DG glycosylation disrupt the binding between α-DG and extracellular matrix ligands, which compromises the muscle cell integrity and leads to dystroglycanopathies (Fig. 2.1.1.1 and Fig. 2.1.1.2) [146].

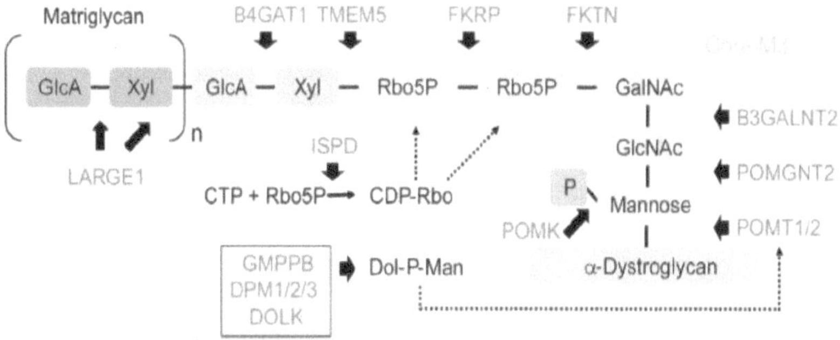

Fig. 2.1.1.1 Enzymes involved in the glycosylation of α-DG Core M3. Blue texts mark the enzymes involved in the glycosylation of α-DG Core M3 and its extension. Functions of these enzymes can be evaluated by the IIH6C4 antibody. Bold arrows link enzymes to the modifications or glycan additions they catalyze; for instance, POMK catalyzes mannose phosphorylation. Dol-P-Man is dolichol phosphate mannose; GlcNAc, N-acetylglucosamine; GalNAc, N-acetylgalactosamine; Rbo5P, ribitol-5-phosphate; Xyl, xylose; GlcA, glucronic acid.

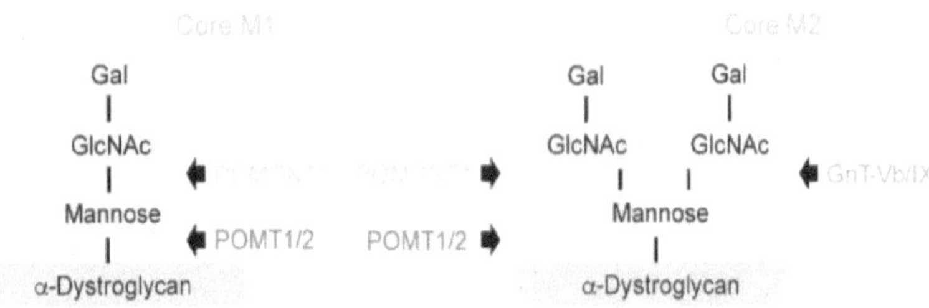

Fig. 2.1.1.2 Enzymes involved in the glycosylation of α-DG Core M1 and M2. POMT1/2 participate the glycosylation of α-DG Core M1, M2 and M3. POMGNT1 mutations in patients manifest the hallmark of reduced IIH6C4 signal. GnT-Vb/IX mutations are not known to alter IIH6C4 signals. GlcNAc is N-acetylglucosamine; Gal, galactose.

Among the enzymes, FKRP adds the second ribitol-5-phosphate (Rbo5P) to the Rbo5P tandem [147] while LARGE1 is responsible for adding the repeated disaccharide units of matriglycan [148]. Both enzymes are associated with many rare disease cases, for which novel treatments are being developed vigorously, including new drugs [149], gene therapies [150,151] and cell therapies [152]. This further emphasizes the need for improved variant interpretation to facilitate the enrollment of more patients in these gene-specific trials. However, most variants of α-DG glycosylation enzymes, including FKRP and LARGE1, lack clinical reports and those reported remain poorly interpreted (Fig. 2.1.1.3), with many unique to the families [153]. Despite the recent advancements in population studies [154-157], the challenges associated with comprehensively understanding recessive variants persist, calling for the implementation of DMS.

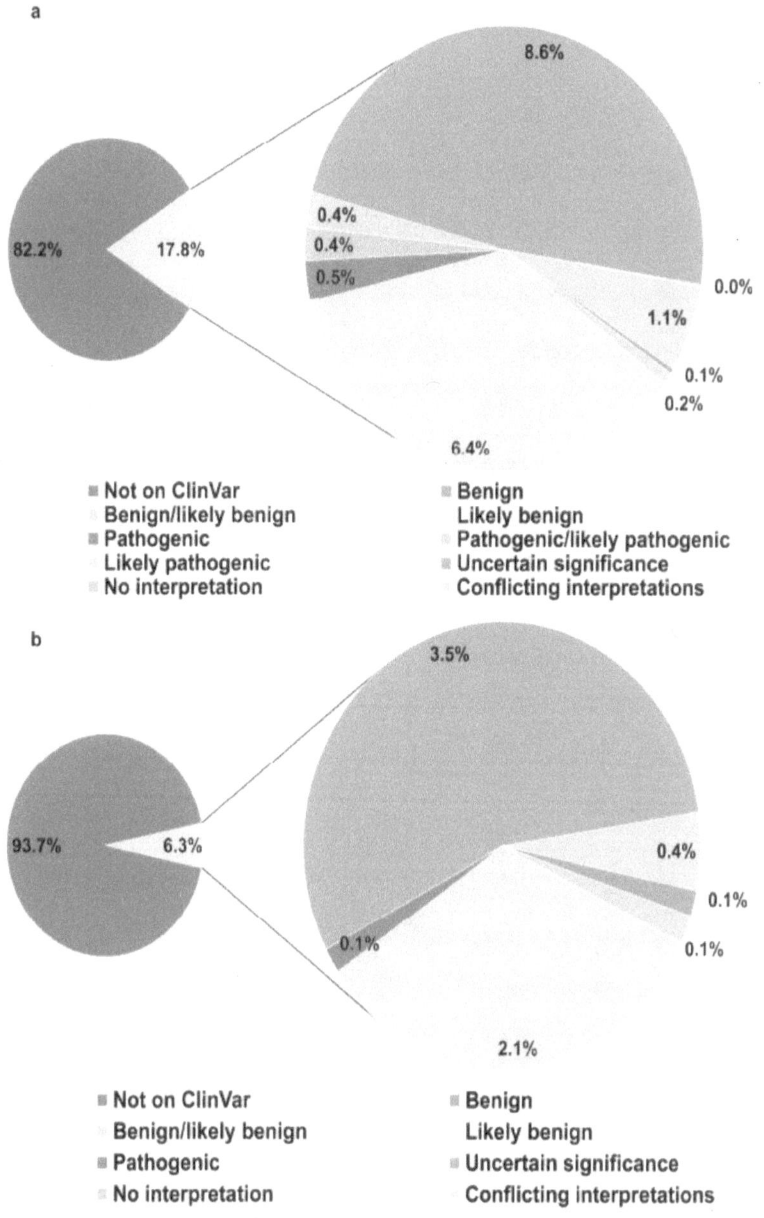

Fig. 2.1.1.3 Limited SNVs in ClinVar were explicitly defined. Most of all possible coding SNVs of α-DG

glycosylation enzyme-coding genes lack clinical reports. Around half (or more) of the SNVs of these genes in ClinVar (April 20, 2023) were classified as variants of uncertain significance. **a**, *FKRP*. **b**, *LARGE1*.

Hypoglycosylation is a molecular phenotype underlying dystroglycanopathies. The IIH6C4 antibody is widely used for α-DG-related research and is an effective tool for detecting this hallmark in clinical diagnoses. IIH6C4 specifically binds to the matriglycan chain of glycosylated α-DG Core M3, allowing for quantification of α-DG glycosylation levels [158]. Functions of the enzymes involved in α-DG Core M3 glycosylation have been evaluated with IIH6C4 in previous studies, including GMPPB [159], DPM1/2/3 [160], DOLK [161], POMT1/2 [162], POMK [163], POMGNT2 [164], B3GALNT2 [165], ISPD [166], FKTN [167], FKRP [168], TMEM5 [169], B4GAT1 [170], and LARGE1 [171] (Fig. 2.1.1.1).

Intriguingly, while variants of GnT-Vb/IX, an enzyme participates in the glycosylation of Core M2, are unlikely to alter IIH6C4 signal [172], variants of POMGNT1, an enzyme that mainly participates in the glycosylation of Core M1 and M2, can perturb the IIH6C4 signal [158] (Fig. 2.1.1.2), potentially by serving as an "enzymatic chaperone" for FKTN [173-176].

Fibroblasts from patients with dystroglycanopathies have been characterized using the IIH6C4 antibody in a fluorescence flow cytometry (FFC) assay [177]. The human haploid cell line, HAP1, has become a widely utilized platform in α-DG-related research, covering various areas such as dystroglycanopathy gene discovery [178], enzymatic functions [163], and α-DG binding properties and functions [179]. Additionally, previous studies have established the compatibility of HAP1 cells with FFC [180]. Building upon these previous studies, we adapted the IIH6C4 FFC assay developed for fibroblasts to be applicable to

HAP1 cells. Through this adaptation, we also increased the sensitivity of the assay, enabling the discrimination of differences between variants (Fig. 2.1.1.4a,b).

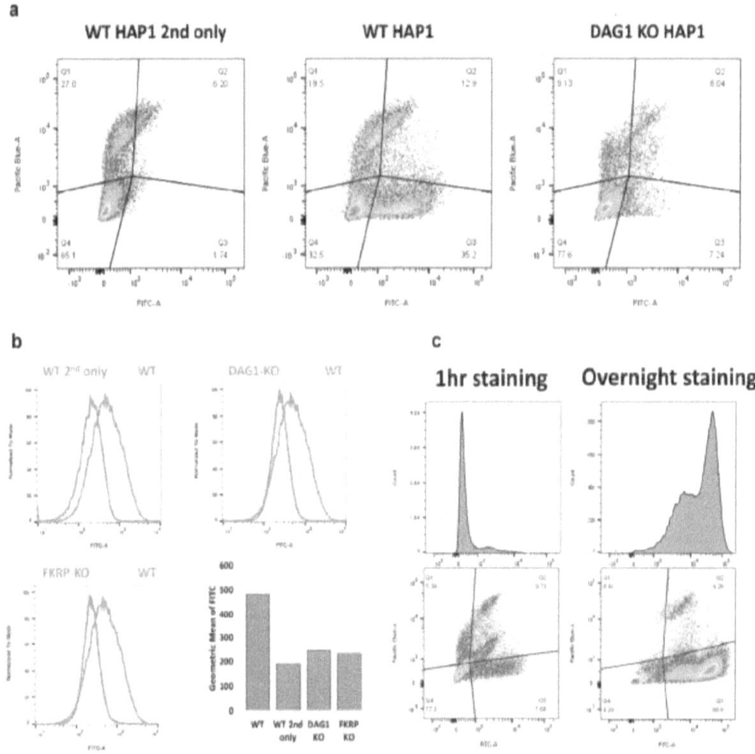

Fig. 2.1.1.4 The IIH6C4 FFC assay and the optimized FACS in the HAP1 platform. Wildtype HAP1 cells and *DAG1*-KO HAP1 cells were ordered from Horizon Discovery. The *DAG1*-KO HAP1 carries a 1-bp deletion (c.205Gdel). *FKRP*-KO HAP1 was established from a single clone of CRISPR RNP nucleofected cells and carries a 1-bp insertion (c.181Adup). **a,b**, IIH6C4 FFC is compatible with the HAP1 platform. 1-hr room temperature staining was performed for both primary and secondary antibodies. (**a**) and (**b**) were two independent experiments. **b**, 1-hr staining is not sensitive enough for a high-throughput FACS-based variant characterization, as the separation between positive signal and null signal is unsatisfactory. **c**, Optimized 4 °C overnight staining increased the assay sensitivity. Both staining protocols used the same samples: Lenti-*DAG1 FKRP*-KO HAP1 rescued by a mixture of Lenti-EF1α-*FKRP* and Lenti-EF1α-*FKRP*(c.826C>A).

The IIH6C4 FFC assay provided a great opportunity for us to improve variant interpretation of the α-DG glycosylation enzymes in a robust and scalable manner and meet both the needs in genetic testing and the diagnostic needs for novel trials. Building upon this assay, we developed a universal DMS workflow called Saturation Mutagenesis-Reinforced Functional Assays (SMuRF) (Fig. 2.1.1.5), and we employed SMuRF to generate functional sores for all possible coding SNVs of FKRP and LARGE1.

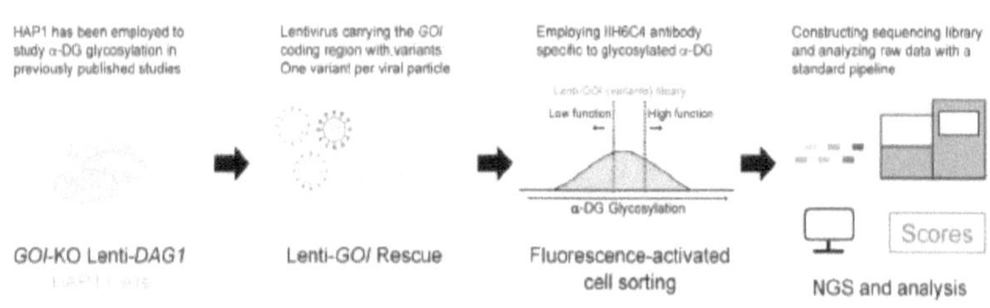

Fig. 2.1.1.5 A universal workflow of SMuRF. SMuRF accompanies saturation mutagenesis with functional assays. Here, the saturation mutagenesis is achieved by delivering variant lentiviral particles to the engineered HAP1 platform where the endogenous gene of interest (GOI) was knocked-out and stable *DAG1* overexpression was established through lentiviral integration. A fluorescence-activated cell sorting (FACS) assay was employed to separate the high function population and the low function population.

2.1.2 Establishing the SMuRF workflow

SMuRF was developed with the aim of creating a universal DMS workflow that is adaptable for various genes by employing appropriate assays. Initially, it was established to characterize all possible coding SNVs for FKRP by employing the IIH6C4-based flow cytometric assay, and subsequently, its adaptability to all α-DG core M3 glycosylation enzymes was demonstrated by its application to LARGE1. The established IIH6C4 SMuRF workflow has 4 major steps:

(1) Establishing engineered cell line platforms. The endogenous gene of interest (GOI), specifically *FKRP* or *LARGE1*, was knocked-out to make *GOI*-KO HAP1 lines (Fig. 2.1.2.1a,b). *DAG1* overexpression was achieved by Lenti-*DAG1* transduction (Fig. 2.1.2.1c-e). Subsequent experiments were performed using monoclonal *GOI*-KO Lenti-*DAG1* HAP1 lines.

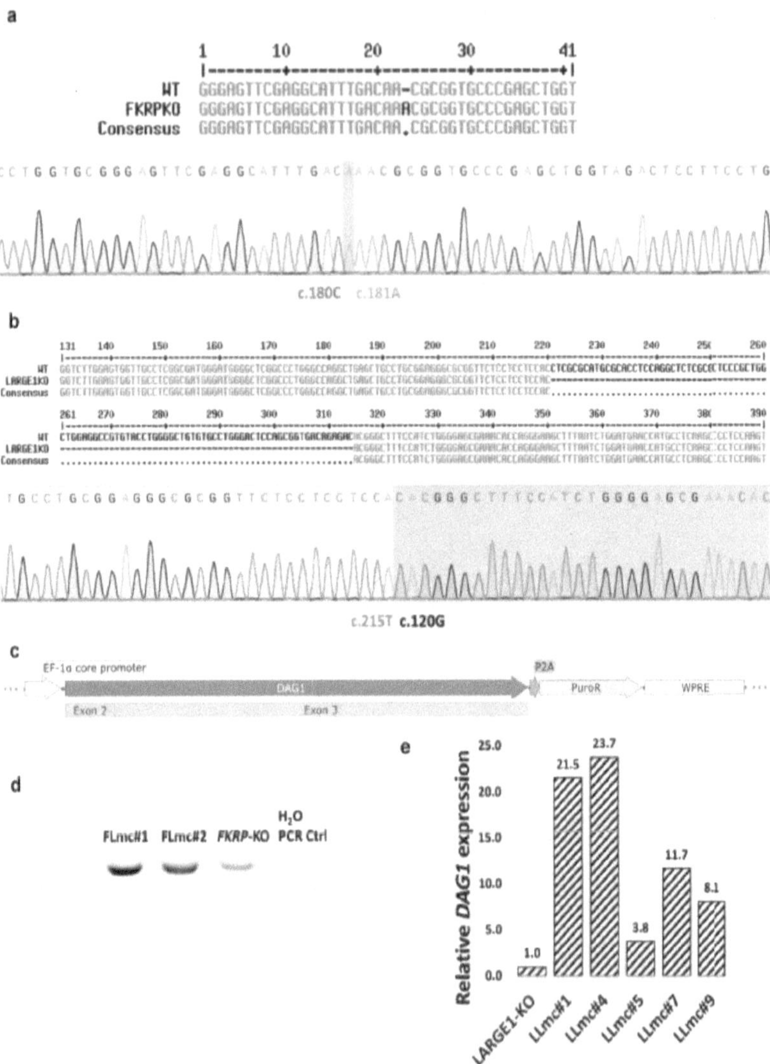

Fig. 2.1.2.1 Create the monoclonal *GOI*-KO Lenti-*DAG1* HAP1 platform cell lines. *GOI*-KO HAP1 monoclonal cell lines were isolated from pooled CRISPR RNP nucleofected cells. **a**, *FKRP*-KO HAP1 carries a 1-bp frameshifting insertion (c.181Adup). **b**, *LARGE1*-KO HAP1 carries a 94-bp frameshifting deletion (c.121_214del). The mutations were validated with Sanger sequencing. α-DG overexpression was achieved with Lenti-*DAG1*. **c**, The Lenti-*DAG1* expression cassette. PuroR was linked to the *DAG1* CDS via a P2A sequence. **d**, RT-PCR experiment for *FKRP*-KO Lenti-*DAG1* monoclonal lines (FLmc#1 and FLmc#2). Same amount of RNA molecules was used for each reaction. Bands in lane 2-5 were the PCR products of the *DAG1* cDNA primers (225 bp). Bands in lane 1&6 were 200-bp ladder bands.

FLmc#1 was chosen as the cell line platform for downstream experiments. **e**, RT-qCR experiment for *LARGE1*-KO Lenti-*DAG1* monoclonal lines. *HPRT1* primers were used as the housekeeping control for the ddCt quantification. The expression level was normalized to the *LARGE1*-KO sample. qPCR triplicates were set for each condition. LLmc#1 was chosen as the cell line platform for downstream experiments.

(2) Creating lentiviral pools of all possible coding SNVs to transduce the platform cells. To accomplish this step, we first constructed the plasmids carrying the wildtype (WT) GOIs. A key consideration here is to employ a weak promoter for the study of enzymatic activity, as over-expression may rescue the pathogenic effects of the low-function variants [181]. We employed a weak promoter UbC for GOI expression [182], creating Lenti-UbC-*FKRP*-EF1α-*BSD* and Lenti-UbC-*LARGE1*-EF1α-*BSD* (Fig. 2.1.2.2a). *BSD* encodes Blasticidin S deaminase (BSD), which confers blasticidin resistance in transduced cells.

Next, we performed saturation mutagenesis to introduce all possible SNVs using the WT plasmids as templates. Currently, well-established saturation mutagenesis methods include but are not limited to the insertion of variant-carrying tiles [23], multiplex homology-directed repair [24], and reversibly-terminated inosine mutagenesis [25]. However, these methods are usually subjected to one or more of the limitations, including intensive labor requirements, high expenses, disparate variant representation, and limited spanning regions. To address these issues, we developed a 2-way extension cloning method called Programmed Allelic Series with Common procedures (PALS-C), which was adapted from PALS [183]. We managed to achieve saturation mutagenesis without the special reagents and equipment required for PALS or the laborious steps required in a previous optimization for PALS [184], which makes PALS-C simple and accessible to most molecular biological laboratories (Fig. 2.1.2.2b).

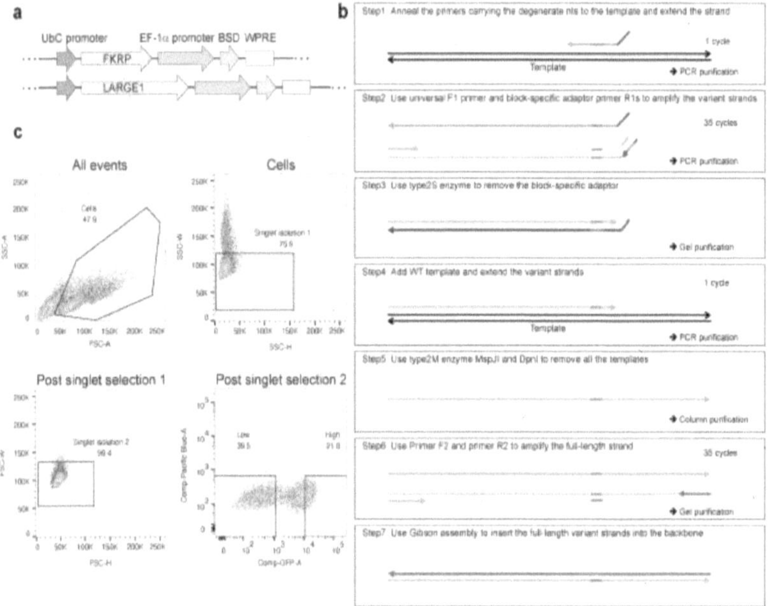

Fig. 2.1.2.2 SMuRF is a universal workflow to characterize SNVs of α-DG glycosylation enzymes. a, Lenti-*GOI* constructs used for the saturation mutagenesis. The *GOI* CDS expression is driven by a weak promoter UbC. **b,** PALS-C is simple and accessible to most molecular biological laboratories. To accommodate the requirements of downstream short-read NGS, the *GOI* variants were separated into multiple blocks (6 blocks for *FKRP* and 10 blocks for *LARGE1*). The PALS-C 2-way extension cloning generates block-specific lentiviral plasmid pools from 1 oligo pool per GOI. The steps are massively multiplexed: Step1 requires only a single-tube reaction; the following steps can be done in a single-tube reaction for each block. **c,** A representative example shows the gating strategy; 20k flow cytometry events of *FKRP* block1 were recorded and reanalyzed with FlowJo.

We adopted a multi-block strategy where we divided the GOI variants into multiple non-overlapping blocks (6 for *FKRP* and 10 for *LARGE1*). For each GOI, PALS-C initiates with one single pool of oligos and eventually generates an isolated lentiviral plasmid pool for each block. All downstream experiments, up to NGS, were conducted individually for each block. This strategy allowed us to employ short-read NGS to examine variant enrichment while avoiding the requirement of an additional

NGS to assign barcodes to variants spanning the entire CDS and the expenses associated with it [185].

Variant representation in the lentiviral plasmid pools generated by PALS-C was evaluated using a shallow NGS service, according to which, more than 99.6% of all possible SNVs were represented (Fig. 2.1.2.3). The plasmid pools were packaged into lentiviral particles, which were subsequently delivered into the platform cells through transduction.

(3) Isolating lentiviral-rescued cells with high or low glycosylation levels through IIH6C4-based fluorescence-activated cell sorting (FACS). Once the transduced cells have undergone drug selection and expanded to an adequate quantity, they can be utilized in FACS. To establish the working conditions for the FACS, staining conditions and gating parameters were tested with mini-libraries to achieve optimized separation of variants with different functional levels (Fig. 2.1.2.4a,b). α-DG glycosylation level was quantified by IIH6C4-FITC signal (Fig. 2.1.2.2c and Fig. 2.1.2.4c,d), based on which cells were sorted to the high-glycosylation group and the low-glycosylation group. The FACS events of each group achieved a minimum of ~1000 × coverage.

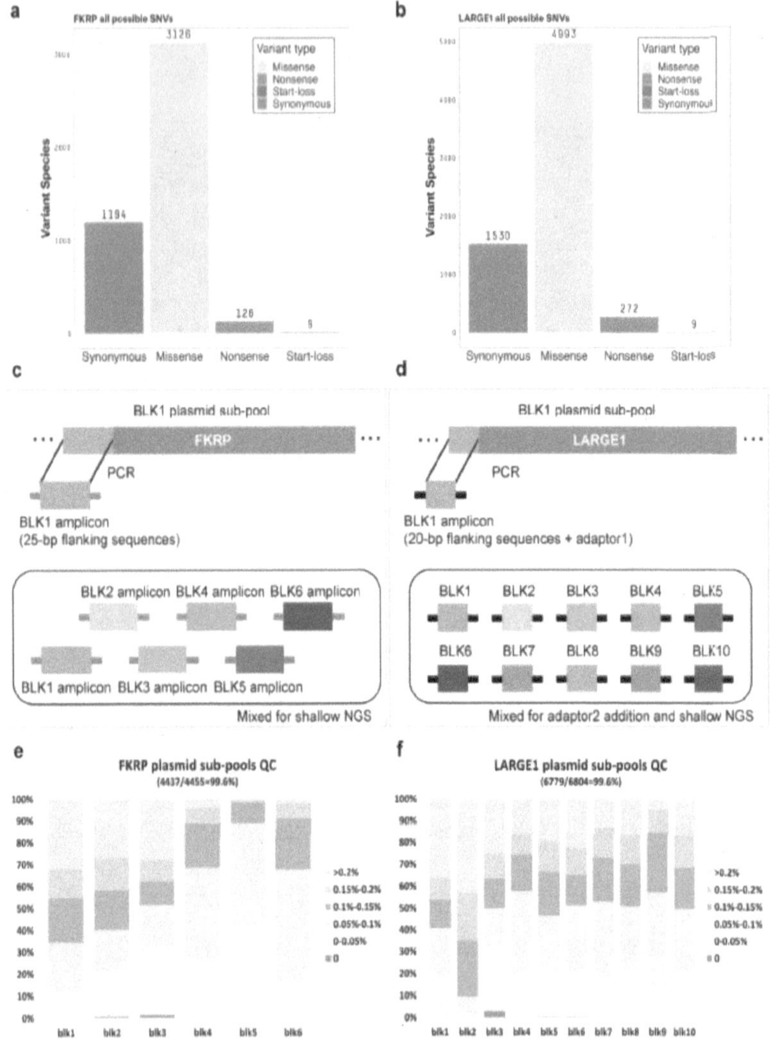

Fig. 2.1.2.3 QC of the lentiviral plasmid pools of *FKRP* and *LARGE1*. We designed and synthesized oligos for all possible CDS SNVs of *FKRP* (**a**) and *LARGE1* (**b**). Stop-loss variants were intentionally excluded from the design due to their incompatibility with the lentivirus-based saturation mutagenesis strategy. Plasmid pool QC was performed using the Amplicon-EZ service. QC sequencing libraries were constructed using PCR amplification strategies for *FKRP* (**c**) and *LARGE1* (**d**). BLK, block. **e,f,** 99.6% of all possible SNVs were represented in the plasmid pools *FKRP* (**e**) and *LARGE1* (**f**). Color groups indicate the variant representation in the pools. If the variants are evenly represented, we expect a 0.13% (FKRP BLK1-5) or a 0.15% (FKRP BLK6; LARGE1 blocks) representation for all variants. Over-representation

suggests co-occurrence of multiple variants on the same lentiviral genomes, which were eventually removed in the analytical pipeline for variant scoring.

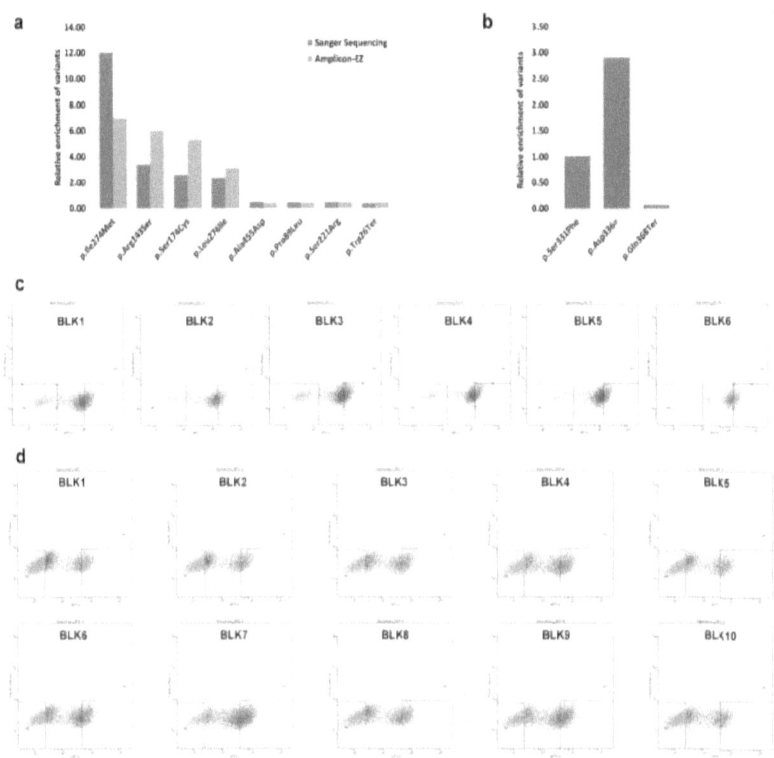

Fig. 2.1.2.4 Optimized FACS assay is capable to separate variants with different function levels. a,b, Mini-libraries were used to optimize the FACS assay to achieve expected separation of variants with known clinical significance; *FKRP* (**a**), *LARGE1* (**b**). Both Amplicon-EZ NGS and Sanger sequencing was used to quantify the variant enrichment for *FKRP*. Sanger sequencing was used to quantify the variant enrichment for *LARGE1*. Relative enrichment was defined as a ratio of a variant's representation in the high-glycosylation group to that in the low-glycosylation group. Higher relative enrichment indicates higher variant function. The *LARGE1* sequence was cloned from HEK293T cDNA. HEK293T carries a heterozygous *LARGE1* mutation (c.1848G>A, p.Met616Ile). This variant was removed when building the *LARGE1* SMuRF lentiviral pools but were kept in this experiment depicted in this figure. Sanger sequencing confirmed the frequency of this mutation in these four lentiviral constructs were: WT 35.1%, S331F 96.3%, D336= 2.0%, Q368*=2.0%. **c,d,** The high-glycosylation group (top ~20%) and low-glycosylation group (bottom ~40%) were gated based on the IIH6C4+FITC signal. Examples shows the FACS gating parameters for all blocks of *FKRP* (**c**) and *LARGE1* (**d**). 20k events were recorded. Cell debris and multiplets were pre-excluded before the sorting.

(4) Building the NGS library and generating the SMuRF scores. Genome DNA from each group of each block was used to build the sequencing library using a 3-round PCR strategy (Fig. 2.1.2.5a). Raw NGS datasets were analyzed with our customized workflow Gargamel-Azrael to generate SMuRF scores for all variants (Fig. 2.1.2.5b). Essentially, SMuRF score is the normalized relative enrichment of a variant in the FACS groups (2.3). High SMuRF scores indicate high function of variants to glycosylate α-DG while low scores indicate low function. Two transduction replicates were performed for *FKRP* to confirm the reproducibility of the workflow (Fig. 2.1.2.6).

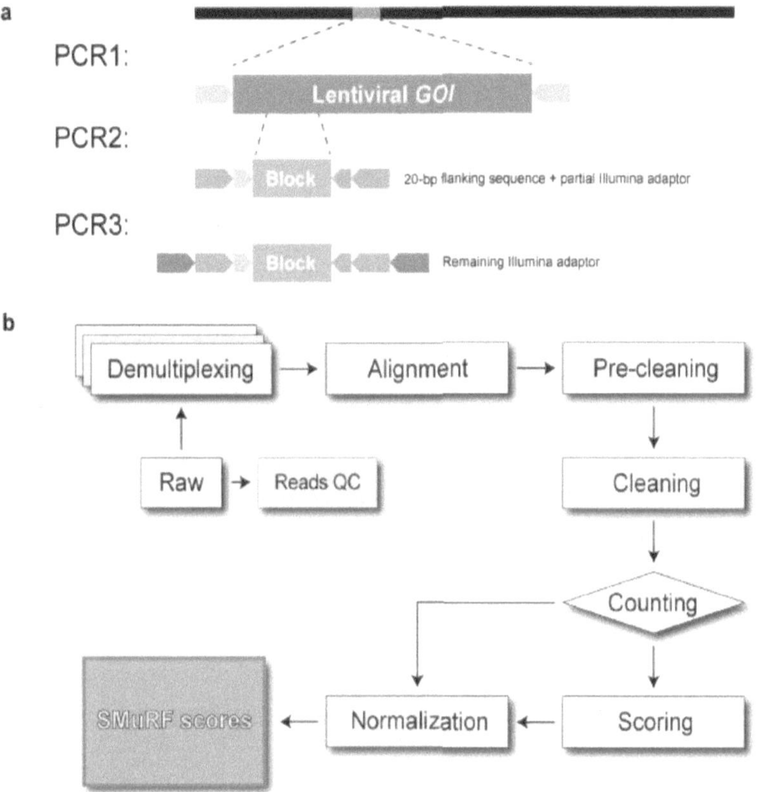

Fig. 2.1.2.5 Building the NGS library and generating the SMuRF scores. Genome DNA was extracted from each group of each block. **a**, A 3-round PCR strategy to build the NGS library. Samples from the high and low glycosylation groups were barcoded differently in PCR2. PCR2 products of all samples were multiplexed for a single PCR3 reaction. **b**, a universal pipeline to generate SMuRF scores from raw NGS data. Steps colored with yellow indicate employment of customized scripts. Cleaning is a critical step where the reads carrying co-occurred variants are filtered out. Alignment, pre-cleaning, cleaning and counting were performed with scripts in the Gargamel repository; scoring, normalization and downstream plotting were performed with scripts in the Azrael repository.

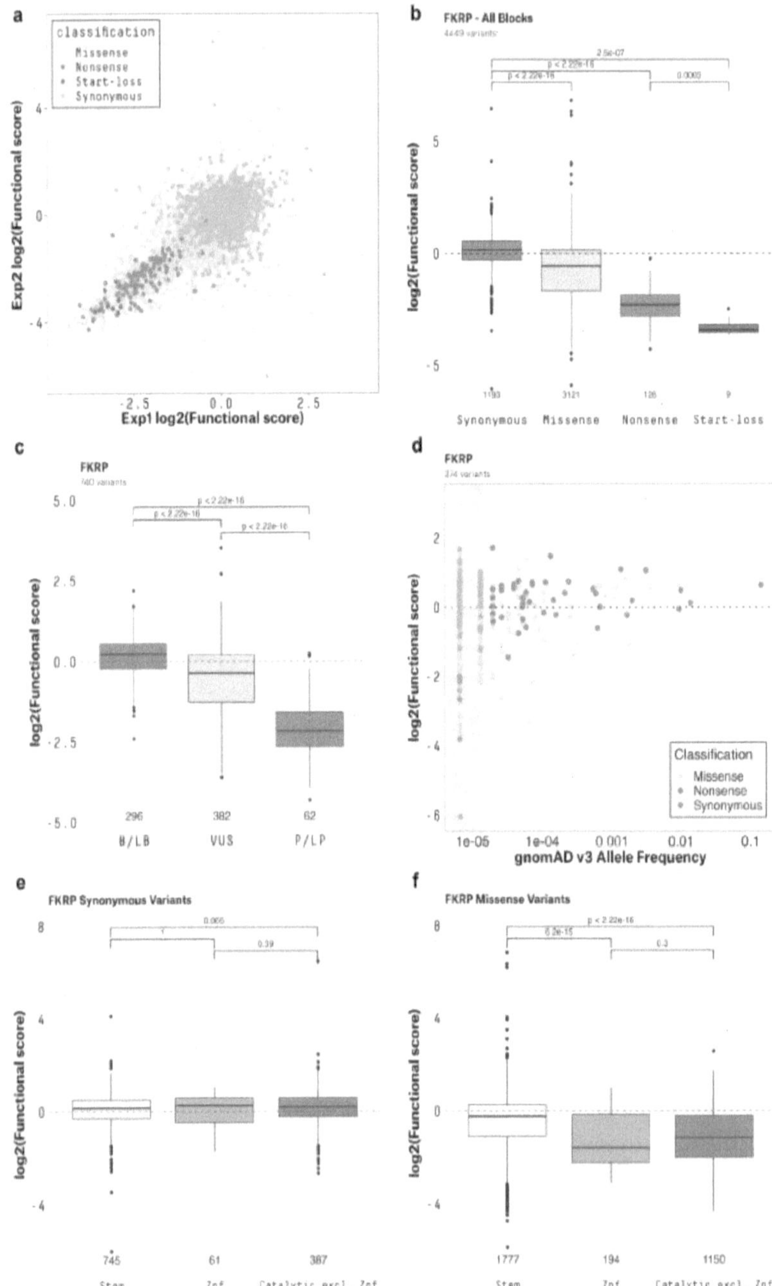
a
classification
Missense
Nonsense
Start-loss
Synonymous
Exp2 log2(Functional score)
Exp1 log2(Functional score)
b
FKRP - All Blocks
4449 variants
log2(Functional score)
Synonymous
Missense
Nonsense
Start-loss
c
FKRP
740 variants
log2(Functional score)
B/LB
VUS
P/LP
d
FKRP
log2(Functional score)
Classification
Missense
Nonsense
Synonymous
gnomAD v3 Allele Frequency
e
FKRP Synonymous Variants
log2(Functional score)
Stem
Znf
Catalytic excl. Znf
f
FKRP Missense Variants
log2(Functional score)
Stem
Znf
Catalytic excl. Znf

Fig. 2.1.2.6 Two transduction replicates for FKRP confirmed the reproducibility of SMuRF. Two transduction replicates, Exp1 and Exp2, were performed for FKRP using the same protocol. Exp1 utilized a commercial IIH6C4 antibody (Sigma-Aldrich, 05-593, discontinued), while Exp2 utilized an in-house IIH6C4 antibody from Dr. Kevin Campbell's lab. The results of Exp1 are presented in the section below. **a,** The SMuRF scores from these two experiments exhibited a good correlation. The Spearman's rank correlation rho is 0.66. **b-f,** Exp2 exhibited the same patterns as Exp1 in terms of variant types, ClinVar classification, gnomAD allele frequency (AF), and structural features. Box plots depict the 25th/75th percentiles (box boundaries), median (horizontal line), and an additional 1.5 times IQR (vertical line) above and below the box boundaries. p-values were calculated using the two-sided Wilcoxon test. Counts of variants were labeled below the boxes. **b-f:** dashed lines represent WT functional score.

2.2 Application of SMuRF in FKRP and LARGE1

2.2.1 SMuRF recapitulated and expanded the knowledge gained from population databases

SMuRF scores were generated for ~99.9% of all possible coding SNVs of *FKRP* (4450/4455) and 100% of *LARGE1* (6804/6804). The variants missing from the *FKRP* pools were: c.279G>C, c.430A>C, c.432G>C, c.439G>C and c.454A>C.

SMuRF scores align with the anticipated patterns of different variant types (Fig. 2.2.1.1a,b). The SMuRF score of the WT was set to 0. The synonymous variants display scores that closely approximate the WT score, exhibiting a narrow range of values. *FKRP* synonymous variants have a median of 0.17, with a 95% confidence interval (CI) of 0.14~0.21, while *LARGE1* synonymous variants have a median of 0.20 (95% CI: 0.16~0.24).

The nonsense variants consistently exhibit low SMuRF scores, with sparse outliers observed. *FKRP* nonsense variants have a median of -2.27 (95% CI: -2.42~-2.17), while *LARGE1* nonsense variants have a median of -2.02 (95% CI: -2.11~-1.93). Two noteworthy outliers among the nonsense variants are *FKRP* c.1477G>T (p.Gly493Ter) (SMuRF=-0.42) and *LARGE1* c.2257G>T (p.Glu753Ter)

(SMuRF=0.04). These two are the nonsense variants positioned closest possible to their respective canonical stop codons. The relatively high SMuRF scores of these two variants suggest that their impact on the enzymatic function is negligible in the context of the CDS constructs. Furthermore, since both variants are in the last exon of their respective transcripts, it is also unlikely for them to be substantially influenced by nonsense-mediated decay (NMD) [186].

Notably, the start-loss variants exhibit markedly low SMuRF scores, significantly lower than those observed in most nonsense variants (p-value=9.2e-5, *FKRP*; 0.0034, *LARGE1*). *FKRP* start-loss variants have a median of -3.09 (95% CI: -3.47~-2.93), while *LARGE1* start-loss variants have a median of -2.55 (95% CI: -2.93~-2.25). This observation indicates that, at least in the context of the *FKRP* and *LARGE1* SMuRF CDS constructs, there is a lack of effective genetic compensation to counter the start-loss variants, such as functional downstream alternative start codons [187]. The homozygous start-loss variant *FKRP* c.1A>G (SMuRF=-3.31) has been reported to be associated with WWS, the most severe FKRP-related disorder. This variant has been documented in two cases, with one resulting in the unfortunate death of a child at the age of 6 days and the other leading to a terminated pregnancy [144]. The multi-exon CDS structure of *LARGE1* may confer genetic compensations for start-loss variants that are undetectable by SMuRF [188]. However, in the case of *FKRP*, where there is only one coding exon, the SMuRF scores effectively indicate that start-loss variants pose a high risk of being highly damaging. Therefore, these variants warrant increased attention in genetic testing protocols.

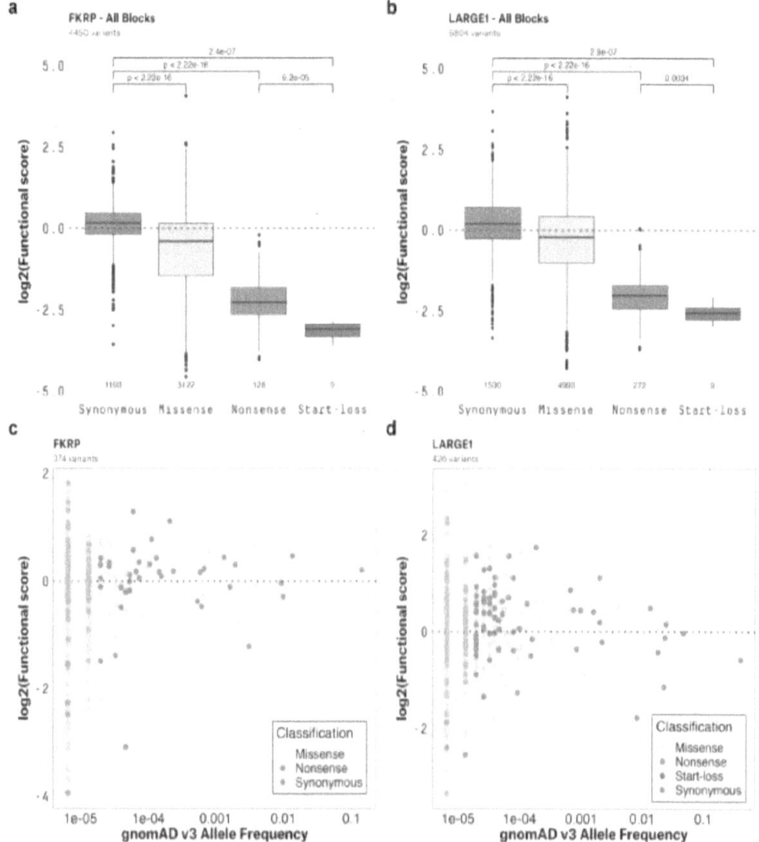

Fig. 2.2.1.1 SMuRF recapitulated and expended the knowledge gained from population databases. SMuRF scores align with variant types (**a**, *FKRP*; **b**, *LARGE1*): synonymous variants resemble wildtype, nonsense variants consistently have low scores, and start-loss variants exhibit markedly lower scores than nonsense variants. Noteworthy outliers include high-scoring nonsense variants at the end of coding sequences. The box boundaries represent the 25th/75th percentiles, with a horizontal line indicating the median and a vertical line marking an additional 1.5 times interquartile range (IQR) above and below the box boundaries. p-values were calculated using the two-sided Wilcoxon test. Counts of variants were labeled below the boxes. SMuRF revealed functional constraints based on variants reported in gnomAD v3.1.2 (**c**, *FKRP*; **d**, *LARGE1*): Low allele frequency variants had diverse functional scores, while high allele frequency variants converged towards wildtype due to selection pressures (Gray box: Allele Count=1 or 2). **a-d**: dashed lines represent WT functional score.

Allele frequency refers to the relative frequency of a genetic variant at a specific chromosomal locus within a population. When combined with allele frequency data obtained from population databases, SMuRF scores were consistent with the selection against pathogenic variants. The Genome Aggregation Database (gnomAD) is a resource that aggregated and harmonized both exome and genome sequencing data from a wide variety of large-scale sequencing projects [189]. The SMuRF scores of the *FKRP* and *LARGE1* variants reported in the large population database gnomAD v3.1.2 [190] were examined. Low allele frequency variants (Allele count= 1 or 2) exhibited a wide range of functional scores, while variants with higher frequency showed functional scores converging towards the WT score due to the selective exclusion of pathogenic variants from the population (Fig. 2.2.1.1c,d). As one of the largest population databases, gnomAD currently provides reports for only 374 *FKRP* coding SNVs (8.4%) and 426 *LARGE1* coding SNVs (6.3%). The ability of SMuRF scores to recapitulate the patterns observed in gnomAD makes them a significant expansion to gnomAD.

The α-DG glycoepitope, as well as the enzymes involved in its glycosylation, are largely conserved within Metazoa. Orthologous sequence similarities of both human *FKRP* and *LARGE1* can be identified in organisms as primitive as choanoflagellates [173]. Evolutionary conservation scores, such as PhyloP scores, indicate the degree of conservation of a variant derived from multiple sequence alignments across species [191]. When compared with PhyloP scores calculated from 100 vertebrates, SMuRF demonstrated the evolutionary tolerance of relatively harmless variants and the selection against damaging variants in both *FKRP* and *LARGE1* (Fig. 2.2.1.2), with a tendency for missense variants to be more disruptive at the more conserved sites (Spearman's rho=-0.38, *FKRP*; -0.21, *LARGE1*).

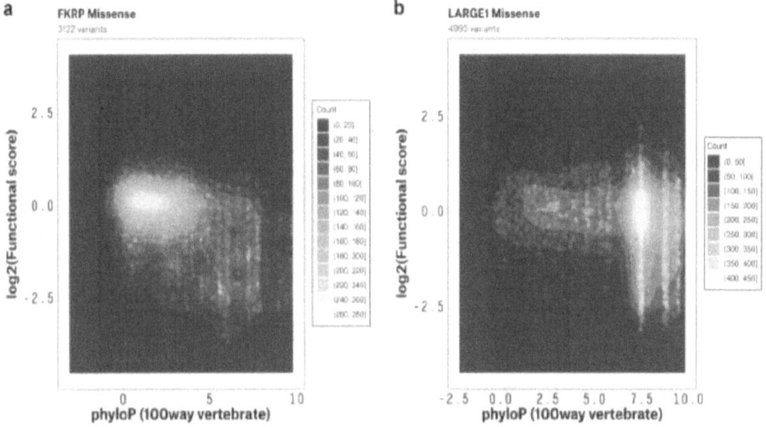

Fig. 2.2.1.2 SMuRF recapitulated the evolutionary selection in both *FKRP* and *LARGE1*. SMuRF scores were compared with the phyloP score calculated from multiple alignments of 100 vertebrate species (**a**, *FKRP*; **b**, *LARGE1*). The higher the phyloP score is, the more conserved a genomic site is. The missense variants show clustering around the WT SMuRF score (0) at less conserved sites, while they tend to be more disruptive at more conserved sites. Interestingly, the genomic sites of WT-like missense variants are more conserved in *LARGE1* compared to *FKRP*, suggesting a possibility that *LARGE1* might have undergone an additional selection process that is independent of α-DG glycosylation [192-195].

2.2.2 SMuRF improved the scope of clinical interpretation of rare variants and provided good training datasets for computational predictors

ClinVar is a public archive of reports of human variants [196], where the variants were classified according to clinical supporting evidence into different categories including: Benign(B), Benign/likely benign (B/LB), Likely benign(LB), Pathogenic(P), Pathogenic /likely pathogenic (P/LP), Likely pathogenic (LP), and Variants of Uncertain Significance (VUS). SMuRF scores correlate well with clinical classification in ClinVar, with B, B/LB, and LB variants having scores close to the WT score while P, P/LP, and LP variants having low scores (Fig. 2.2.2.1a,b and Fig. 2.2.2.2a,b)

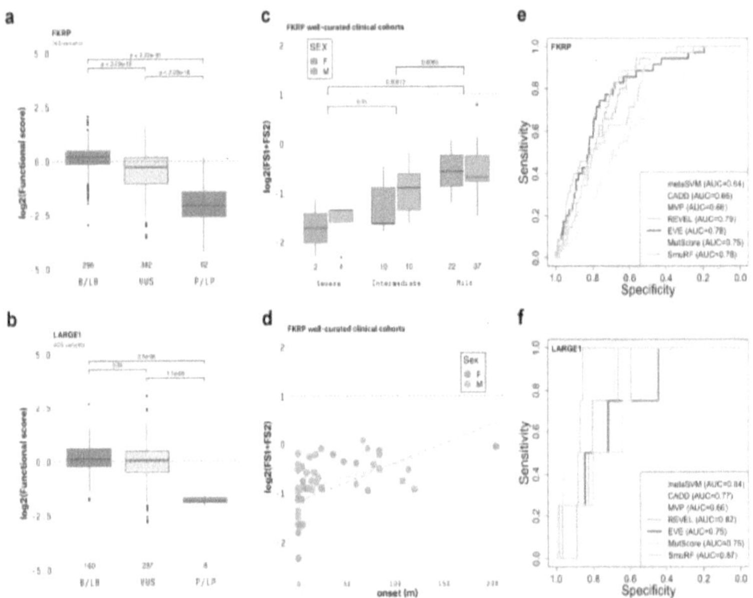

Fig. 2.2.2.1 SMuRF improved the scope of clinical interpretation of rare variants. SMuRF scores correlate well with clinical classification in ClinVar (**a**, *FKRP*; **b**, *LARGE1*). (B/LB: Benign, Benign/Likely benign or Likely benign in ClinVar; VUS: Uncertain significance in ClinVar; P/LP: Pathogenic, Pathogenic/Likely pathogenic or Likely pathogenic in ClinVar.) Counts of variants were labeled below the boxes. Real patient data from eight well-curated cohorts demonstrated that SMuRF scores have the potential to predict disease severity. **c**, The SMuRF scores of variants associated with mild cases were significantly higher than those of intermediate and severe cases. Counts of cases were labeled below the boxes. **a-c**: Box plots depict the 25th/75th percentiles (box boundaries), median (horizontal line), and an additional 1.5 times IQR (vertical line) above and below the box boundaries. p-values were calculated using the Wilcoxon test. **d**, The SMuRF scores are correlated with the disease onset age. Dashed trendlines represent linear regression. Spearman's rank correlation rho: 0.61 (all data), 0.48 (male), 0.77 (female). **c,d**: FS1, the functional score of the variant on Allele1; FS2, the functional score of the variant on Allele2. **a-d**: blue dashed lines represent (homozygous) WT functional score. SMuRF demonstrated high performance in accurately classifying pathogenic variants. Receiver operating characteristic (ROC) curves of SMuRF and computational predictors: taking Pathogenic, Pathogenic/Likely pathogenic and Likely pathogenic variants in ClinVar as true positives (**e**, *FKRP*; **f**, *LARGE1*). AUC: Area Under Curve. Higher AUC indicates better performance in classifying pathogenic variants.

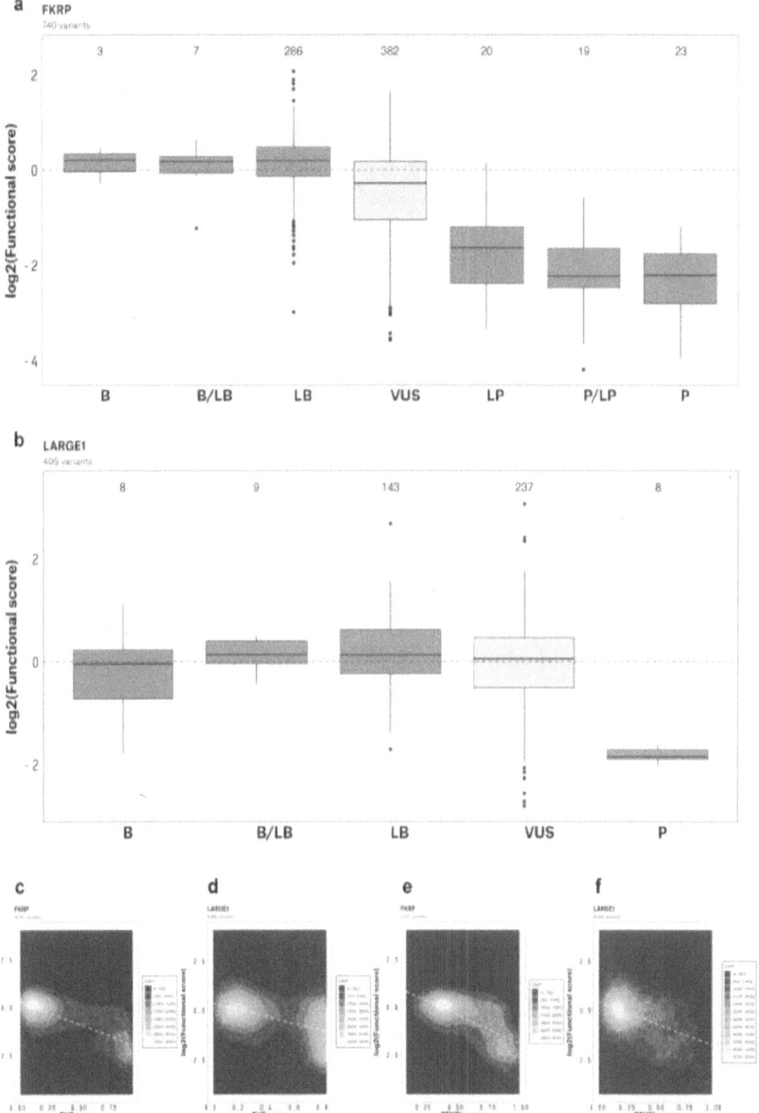

Fig. 2.2.2.2 SMuRF expanded the scope of clinical interpretation for rare variants and provided robust training datasets for computational predictors. SMuRF scores correlate well with clinical classification in ClinVar (**a**, *FKRP*; **b**, *LARGE1*). B: Benign; B/LB: Benign/Likely benign; LB: Likely Benign; P: Pathogenic; P/LP: Pathogenic/Likely pathogenic; LP: Likely pathogenic; VUS: Uncertain significance. Counts of variants were labeled above the boxes. **a**,**b**: Dashed lines represent WT functional score. Among the predictors, EVE has the highest Spearman's coefficient with SMuRF: **c**, -0.62, *FKRP*; **d**, -0.41, *LARGE1*. REVEL demonstrated the best performance according to the ROC curves (Fig. 2.2.2.1e,f), and

also exhibited high Spearman's coefficient with SMuRF: e, -0.58, *FKRP*; f, -0.39, *LARGE1*. White dashed lines represent linear regression.

Furthermore, dystroglycanopathies encompass a spectrum of diseases with varying severity, including severe cases like WWS and muscle-eye-brain disease (MEB), intermediate cases like congenital muscular dystrophies (CMD), and relatively mild cases like LGMDR9 (LGMD2I) [141,144]. We wanted to examine whether SMuRF scores could be used to predict the severity of a variant. We employed a naive additive model where the functional scores of the variants on both alleles were combined through addition to calculate the biallelic functional score. Initially, we conducted the analysis using the disease conditions reported in ClinVar, but no significant pattern was observed (Fig. 2.2.2.3). We believe this is likely due to the suboptimal accuracy in the ClinVar reports. We came to realize that well-curated reports are essential for such analysis. Hence, we aggregated data from 8 well-curated cohorts and compared them with SMuRF scores [144,145,168,197-201]. The functional scores of the variants associated with mild cases were significantly higher compared to those of the intermediate and severe cases (Fig. 2.2.2.1c). Additionally, SMuRF scores showed a correlation with the reported disease onset age (Fig. 2.2.2.1d), where high-function variants were associated with later onset (Spearman's rho=0.61; 0.48, male; 0.77, female).

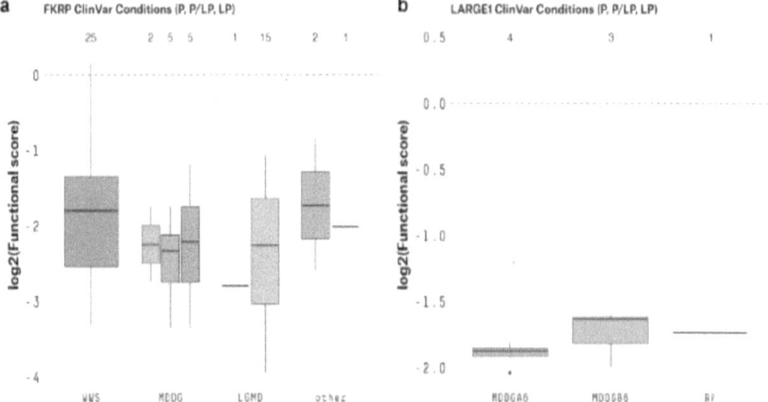

Fig. 2.2.2.3 The accuracy of the disease conditions reported in ClinVar was suboptimal. The SMuRF scores of variants classified as Pathogenic (P), Pathogenic/Likely Pathogenic (P/LP), and Likely Pathogenic (LP) in ClinVar did not show a significant pattern when grouped according to the reported conditions in ClinVar. (**a**, *FKRP*; **b**, *LARGE1*). WWS: Walker-Warburg syndrome. MDDG: muscular dystrophy dystroglycanopathies (left to right: type A1, type A5, type B5). LGMD: limb girdle muscular dystrophy (left to right: not specified; type R9/2I). Other: not specified (left to right: Abnormality of the musculature, Cardiovascular phenotype). RP: retinitis pigmentosa. Box plots depict the 25th/75th percentiles (box boundaries), median (horizontal line), and an additional 1.5 times IQR (vertical line) above and below the box boundaries. Counts of cases were labeled above the boxes. Blue dashed line represents WT functional score.

These analyses above indicate the potential utility of the SMuRF scores for improving variant interpretation. The SMuRF scores can be used to aid in the classification of VUSs and improve the interpretation of LP and LB variants. Additionally, the knowledge gained from well-curated reports can be used to predict the severity of the variants. However, it is important to acknowledge the presence of technical outliers in the SMuRF scores, which primarily arise from inherent limitations of PALS-C and coverage issues in the FACS method. To enhance credibility, we have introduced confidence scores in the reclassification process (Table 2.2.2.4, 2.2.2.5 and Fig. 2.2.2.6, 2.2.2.7). Our ultimate goal is to utilize SMuRF reclassification as an additional line of evidence in clinical variant interpretation, thereby aiding in clinical decision-making.

Clinvar clinical significance	SMuRF reclassification	confidence	Counts
P/LP	SMuRF Benign	High	3
P/LP	SMuRF Benign	Medium	1
P/LP	SMuRF Benign	Low	0
P/LP	SMuRF Mild	High	14
P/LP	SMuRF Mild	Medium	3
P/LP	SMuRF Mild	Low	0
P/LP	SMuRF Intermediate	High	15
P/LP	SMuRF Intermediate	Medium	3
P/LP	SMuRF Intermediate	Low	0
P/LP	SMuRF Severe	High	13
P/LP	SMuRF Severe	Medium	9
P/LP	SMuRF Severe	Low	1
VUS	SMuRF Benign	High	148
VUS	SMuRF Benign	Medium	137
VUS	SMuRF Benign	Low	9
VUS	SMuRF Mild	High	30
VUS	SMuRF Mild	Medium	41
VUS	SMuRF Mild	Low	4
VUS	SMuRF Intermediate	High	17
VUS	SMuRF Intermediate	Medium	9
VUS	SMuRF Intermediate	Low	5
VUS	SMuRF Severe	High	15
VUS	SMuRF Severe	Medium	15
VUS	SMuRF Severe	Low	3
B/LB	SMuRF Benign	High	135
B/LB	SMuRF Benign	Medium	122
B/LB	SMuRF Benign	Low	13
B/LB	SMuRF Mild	High	7
B/LB	SMuRF Mild	Medium	14
B/LB	SMuRF Mild	Low	2
B/LB	SMuRF Intermediate	High	0
B/LB	SMuRF Intermediate	Medium	2
B/LB	SMuRF Intermediate	Low	0
B/LB	SMuRF Severe	High	1
B/LB	SMuRF Severe	Medium	0
B/LB	SMuRF Severe	Low	0
Unclassified	SMuRF Benign	High	1143
Unclassified	SMuRF Benign	Medium	1144
Unclassified	SMuRF Benign	Low	126
Unclassified	SMuRF Mild	High	321
Unclassified	SMuRF Mild	Medium	258
Unclassified	SMuRF Mild	Low	34
Unclassified	SMuRF Intermediate	High	175
Unclassified	SMuRF Intermediate	Medium	83
Unclassified	SMuRF Intermediate	Low	9
Unclassified	SMuRF Severe	High	190
Unclassified	SMuRF Severe	Medium	159
Unclassified	SMuRF Severe	Low	17

Table 2.2.2.4 A potential SMuRF classification for *FKRP*. SMuRF classification serves as a potential variant classification based on SMuRF scores. However, it is important to note that clinical variant interpretation involves the application of various criteria, and functional data such as SMuRF scores are just one piece of the contributing evidence. ClinVar clinical significance: P/LP: Pathogenic, Pathogenic/Likely pathogenic, and Likely pathogenic; B/LB: Benign, Benign/Likely benign, and Likely Benign; VUS: Uncertain significance, Conflicting interpretations of pathogenicity, and no interpretation for the single variant. Boundary score between SMuRF Benign and SMuRF Mild(B2M) was determined according to the inflection point between the ClinVar P/LP and ClinVar B/LB densities in the density plot. Log2(B2M)=-0.7436399. Boundary score between SMuRF Mild and SMuRF Intermediate (M2I) was determined according to the peak value of the mild cases from the 8 well-curated cohorts in the density plot. Log2(M2I)=-0.7358121-1. Boundary score between SMuRF Intermediate and SMuRF Severe (I2S) was determined according to the peak value of the severe cases from the 8 well-curated cohorts in the density plot. Log2(I2S)=-1.307241-1. The real patient data used naive additive biallelic scores. Here, "-1" was used to calculate the equivalent monoallelic scores.

Clinvar clinical significance	SMuRF reclassification	confidence	Counts
P/LP	SMuRF Benign	High	0
P/LP	SMuRF Benign	Medium	0
P/LP	SMuRF Benign	Low	0
P/LP	SMuRF Pathogenic	High	5
P/LP	SMuRF Pathogenic	Medium	3
P/LP	SMuRF Pathogenic	Low	0
VUS	SMuRF Benign	High	135
VUS	SMuRF Benign	Medium	95
VUS	SMuRF Benign	Low	12
VUS	SMuRF Pathogenic	High	8
VUS	SMuRF Pathogenic	Medium	11
VUS	SMuRF Pathogenic	Low	0
B/LB	SMuRF Benign	High	79
B/LB	SMuRF Benign	Medium	73
B/LB	SMuRF Benign	Low	6
B/LB	SMuRF Pathogenic	High	2
B/LB	SMuRF Pathogenic	Medium	0
B/LB	SMuRF Pathogenic	Low	0
Unclassified	SMuRF Benign	High	2492
Unclassified	SMuRF Benign	Medium	2441
Unclassified	SMuRF Benign	Low	272
Unclassified	SMuRF Pathogenic	High	692
Unclassified	SMuRF Pathogenic	Medium	438
Unclassified	SMuRF Pathogenic	Low	40

Table 2.2.2.5 A potential SMuRF classification for *LARGE1*. SMuRF classification serves as a potential variant classification based on SMuRF scores. However, it is important to note that clinical variant interpretation involves the application of various criteria, and functional data such as SMuRF scores are just one piece of the contributing evidence. ClinVar clinical significance: P/LP: Pathogenic, Pathogenic/Likely pathogenic, and Likely pathogenic; B/LB: Benign, Benign/Likely benign, and Likely Benign; VUS: Uncertain significance, Conflicting interpretations of pathogenicity, and no interpretation for the single variant. Boundary score between SMuRF Benign and SMuRF Pathogenic (B2P) was determined according to the inflection point between the ClinVar P/LP and ClinVar B/LB densities in the density plot. Log2(B2P)=-1.405088.

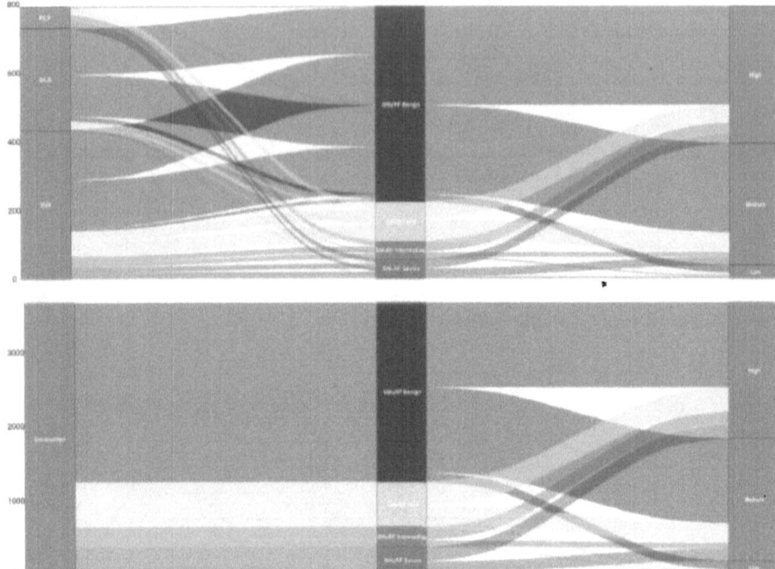

Fig. 2.2.2.6 SMuRF classification and reclassification for *FKRP* variants. ClinVar classified variants were reclassified with SMuRF. (P/LP: Pathogenic, Pathogenic/Likely pathogenic, and Likely pathogenic; B/LB: Benign, Benign/Likely benign, and Likely Benign; VUS: Uncertain significance, Conflicting interpretations of pathogenicity, and no interpretation for the single variant). Previously unclassified variants were classified with SMuRF. Boundary score between SMuRF Benign and SMuRF Mild (B2M) was determined according to the inflection point between the ClinVar P/LP and ClinVar B/LB densities in the density plot. Log2(B2M)=-0.7436399. Boundary score between SMuRF Mild and SMuRF Intermediate (M2I) was determined according to the peak value of the mild cases from the 8 well-curated cohorts in the density plot. Log2(M2I)=-0.7358121-1. Boundary score between SMuRF Intermediate and SMuRF Severe (I2S) was determined according to the peak value of the severe cases from the 8 well-curated cohorts in the density plot. Log2(I2S)=-1.307241-1. The real patient data used naive additive biallelic scores. Here, "-1" was used to calculate the equivalent monoallelic scores.

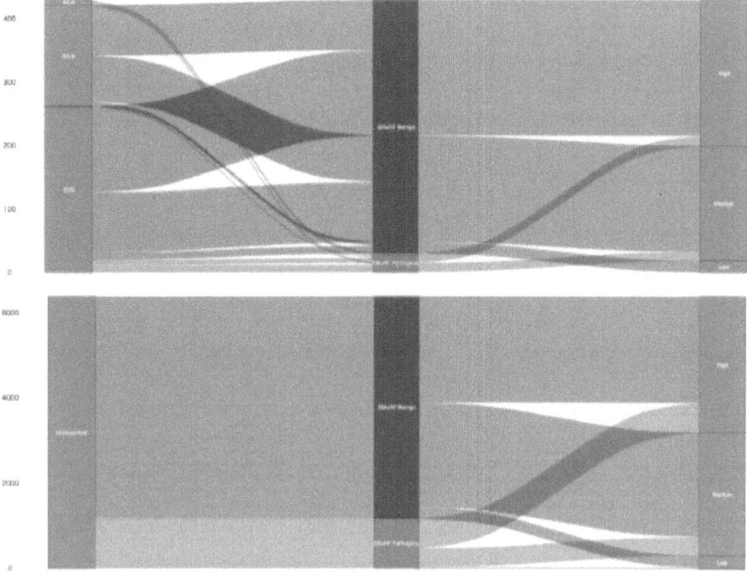

Fig. 2.2.2.7 SMuRF classification and reclassification for *LARGE1* variants. ClinVar classified variants were redassified with SMuRF. (P/LP: Pathogenic, Pathogenic/Likely pathogenic, and Likely pathogenic; B/LB: Benign, Benign/Likely benign, and Likely Benign; VUS: Uncertain significance, Conflicting interpretations of pathogenicity, and no interpretation for the single variant). Previously unclassified variants were classified with SMuRF. Boundary score between SMuRF Benign and SMuRF Pathogenic (B2P) was determined according to the inflection point between the ClinVar P/LP and ClinVar B/LB densities in the density plot. Log2(B2P)=-1.405088.

In addition to assisting in variant re-classification, SMuRF scores can also be used to validate and improve computational predictors. Computational prediction is currently the most scalable and cost-effective method to interpret and predict the functional impact of all novel variants discovered. It is an active area of research with a wealth of methods recently developed, including CADD [202], metaSVM [203], REVEL [204], MVP [205], EVE [206] and MutScore [207]. However, these methods often perform differently depending on the genetic context. To compare SMuRF with these computational predictors, we assessed the receiver operating characteristic (ROC) curves for all methods using the P, P/LP, and

LP variants in ClinVar as true positives (Fig. 2.2.2.1e,f). A higher Area Under Curve (AUC) value indicates better discriminatory ability in classifying pathogenic variants. SMuRF outperforms all computational methods for *LARGE1* (AUC=0.87). For *FKRP*, two predictors, REVEL (AUC=0.79) and EVE (AUC=0.78) exhibit comparable performance to SMuRF (AUC=0.78). We checked the correlation between the predictors and SMuRF. The predictors assigned higher scores to pathogenic variants, hence are negatively correlated with SMuRF scores. EVE scores are derived from an evolutionary model trained with sequences from over 140k species and reported a high concordance with functional assays [206]. Indeed, EVE, among the predictors we tested, has the highest correlation coefficient with SMuRF (Spearman's rho=-0.62, *FKRP*; -0.41, *LARGE1*) (Fig. 2.2.2.2c,d and Table 2.2.2.8). REVEL, among the predictors, demonstrates the best performance according to the ROC curves and also exhibits a relatively good correlation with SMuRF (Spearman's rho=-0.58, *FKRP*; -0.39, *LARGE1*) (Fig. 2.2.2.2e,f). Taken together, these findings demonstrate the potential of SMuRF scores to enhance variant interpretation, both as a standalone line of evidence and in combination with computational predictors.

data	EVE	REVEL	CADD	metaSVM	MVP	MutScore
FKRP-1	-0.6154846	-0.5794562	-0.5035789	-0.3127661	-0.2920998	-0.5786856
LARGE1	-0.4120711	-0.3886374	-0.3350077	-0.3399496	-0.2093022	-0.3918172

Table 2.2.2.8 Spearman's rank correlation rho of SMuRF and the computational predictors.

2.2.3 SMuRF highlighted the critical structural regions

The currently known disease-related mutations in *FKRP* and *LARGE1* are distributed throughout their entire sequences (Fig. 2.2.3.1). As there are only limited known pathogenic variants, no clear pattern has been concluded to identify critical structural regions and associate them to specific disease mechanisms.

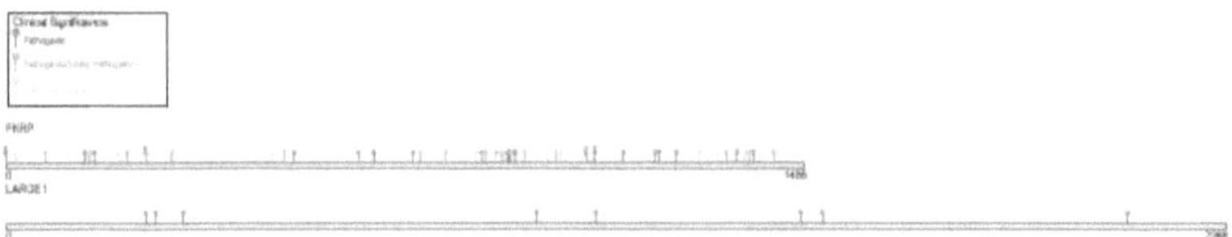

Fig. 2.2.3.1 The currently known disease-related mutations in *FKRP* and *LARGE1* are dispersed throughout their entire sequences. Pathogenic, Pathogenic/Likely pathogenic, and Likely pathogenic variants in ClinVar (April 20, 2023) were labeled at their respective sites on the cDNA sequences.

SMuRF can contribute to highlighting critical structural regions in the enzymes. The protein structures of both FKRP and LARGE1 have been previously studied. FKRP is known to have a stem domain and a catalytic domain [208]. SMuRF scores revealed that missense variants in the catalytic domain are generally more disruptive than those in the stem domain (p-values<2.22e-16) (Fig. 2.2.3.2a). Furthermore, it has been reported that a zinc finger loop within the catalytic domain plays a crucial role in FKRP enzymatic function [208]. SMuRF analysis demonstrated that missense variants in the zinc finger loop exhibit greater disruption compared to variants in the remaining regions of the catalytic domain (p-value=0.0016). The observed differences in the domains are only significant in the case of missense variants, and they are not driven by technical artifacts such as block differences and positional effects as there are no significant differences observed among synonymous variants (p-values>0.1) (Fig. 2.2.3.2b).

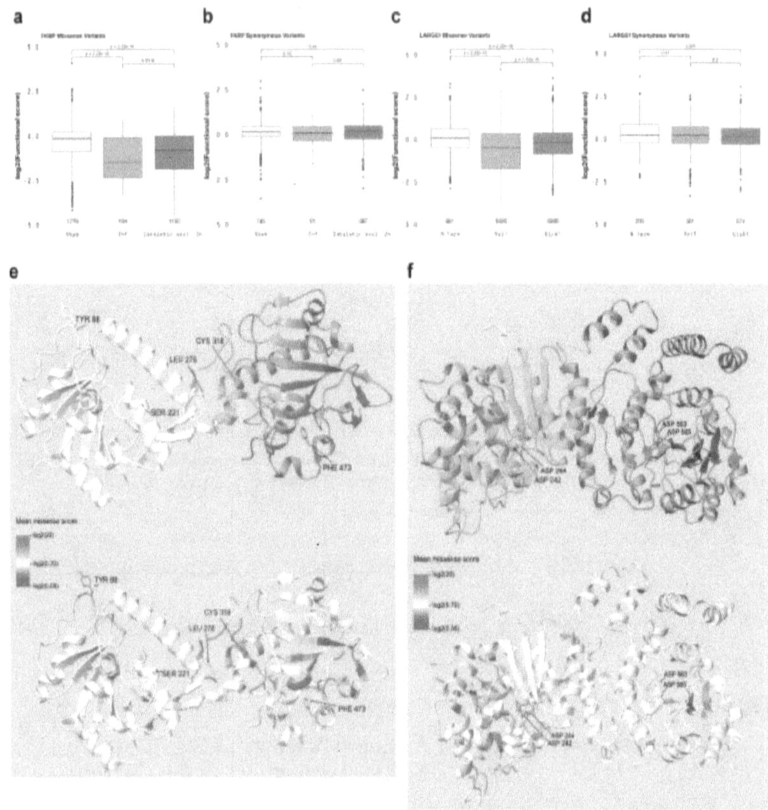

Fig. 2.2.3.2 SMuRF highlighted the critical structural regions. a, SMuRF scores showed higher functional disruption by missense variants in the catalytic domain of *FKRP* compared to the stem domain. The zinc finger loop within the catalytic domain exhibited greater disruption by missense variants. **c,** Missense variants in the catalytic domains of *LARGE1* showed higher disruption compared to the N-terminal domain. Missense variants in the XylT domain were more disruptive than those in the GlcAT domain. The observed domain differences were significant only for missense variants, not synonymous variants (**b,** *FKRP*; **d,** *LARGE1*). Box plots depict the 25th/75th percentiles (box boundaries), median (horizontal line), and an additional 1.5 times IQR (vertical line) above and below the box boundaries. p-values were calculated using the two-sided Wilcoxon test. Counts of variants were labeled below the boxes. Dashed lines represent WT functional score. SMuRF scores were utilized to map SNV-accessible single amino acid substitutions (SNV-SAASs) onto the 3D structures of the enzymes (**e,** *FKRP*; **f,** *LARGE1*). The mean SMuRF score per amino acid residue was calculated and visualized using a color scale, where red indicates positions sensitive to substitutions and green are tolerated. The crystal structure of human FKRP (PDB:6KAM, codon: 45-495) and the electron microscopy structure of LARGE1 (PDB:7UI7, codon: 34-756) were used.

LARGE1 has two catalytic domains: a xylose transferase (XylT) domain and a glucuronate transferase (GlcAT) domain [209]. They are each responsible for adding one unit of the polysaccharide matriglycan chain, which consists of alternating xylose and glucuronate units. SMuRF revealed that the missense variants in both catalytic domains tend to be significantly more disruptive than the variants in the N-terminal domain (p-values<2.22e-16) (Fig. 2.2.3.2c). Interestingly, SMuRF also showed that the variants in the XylT domain tend to be more disruptive than those in the GlcAT domain (p-values<2.22e-16). A previous IIH6C4 western blot experiment revealed a similar observation, demonstrating that mutations deactivating the GlcAT domain, but not the XylT domain, can generate a faint band indicative of glycosylated matriglycan [209]. Together, these observations suggest that the addition of a single xylose to α-DG is sufficient to be detected by IIH6C4, albeit generating a very weak signal. It is uncertain how much physiological function can be achieved by this single xylose in comparison to the complete matriglycan chain. Again, the differences in SMuRF scores between domains were observed exclusively in missense variants and not in synonymous variants (p-values>0.05) (Fig. 2.2.3.2d).

We further mapped the SMuRF scores of SNV-accessible single amino acid substitutions (SNV-SAASs) onto the 3D structures of the enzymes (Fig. 2.2.3.2e,f) (FKRP: PDB 6KAM; LARGE1: PDB 7UI7), thereby highlighting the structural significance of the critical regions. SMuRF confirmed the functional importance of p.Cys318 in FKRP (log2 mean missense =-2.15), which is required for Zn2+ binding in the zinc finger loop [210]. A p.Cys318Tyr variant (SMuRF=-2.12) has been reported to be associated with WWS [200]. SMuRF also highlighted the functional importance of p.Phe473 in FKRP (log2 mean missense =-1.78), which is located in a small hydrophobic pocket essential for CDP-ribitol substrate binding within the catalytic domain [210].

Three important amino acids in the FKRP stem domain were labeled on the 3D structure as well: p.Tyr88 (log2 mean missense =-2.06) and p.Ser221 (log2 mean missense =-0.59), which are situated at the subunit-subunit interface involved in FKRP tetramerization *in vivo*, and p.Leu276 (log2 mean missense =0.35), which interacts with the catalytic domain [208]. P.Tyr88Phe is likely associated with disease [211], and has a low SMuRF score (-3.52). p.Ser221Arg was associated with CMD-MR (MR: mental retardation) [212]. All three p.Ser221Arg SNVs have low SMuRF scores (c.661A>C: -2.13; c.663C>A: -2.21; c.663C>G: -2.18). Moreover, c.663C>A was examined in the mini-library screen and presented low function (Fig. 2.1.2.4a). p.Leu276Ile is a founder mutation in the European population [213], which is commonly associated with milder symptoms [214]. Interestingly, it has a relatively higher SMuRF score (-0.57) and performed more similarly to the benign variants rather than other pathogenic variants in the mini-library screen (Fig. 2.1.2.4a).

In addition, SMuRF highlighted the importance of p.Asp242 (log2 mean missense =-2.20) and p.Asp244 (log2 mean missense =-1.96) in LARGE1, which are crucial for XylT activity, as well as p.Asp563 (log2 mean missense =-0.48) and p.Asp565 (log2 mean missense =-0.55), which are required for GlcAT activity [209].

It is important to note that at a specific amino acid site, SNV-SAASs can involve substitutions from one amino acid to another with similar or different biochemical properties. The co-occurrence of these scenarios can moderate the mean SMuRF score of this site. Finally, variants affecting different enzyme domains may require distinct treatment approaches [215]. SMuRF, by highlighting critical regions in different domains, can assist in selecting appropriate treatments for different variants.

2.2.4 Validations confirmed SMuRF findings in the myogenic context

One caveat of SMuRF is that the HAP1 platform cell line, although widely used in α-DG-related studies, may not fully reflect the clinical relevance of dystroglycanopathies, which primarily affect neuromuscular tissues [216]. To address this issue, we generated a myogenic platform cell line by engineering MB135, a human control myoblast cell line [217]. Endogenous *FKRP* or *LARGE1* were knocked out respectively in the MB135 cell line. Monoclonal lines were established for both genes (Fig. 2.2.4.1a). Despite being incompatible with the flow cytometric assay (Fig. 2.2.4.1c), the KO MB135 myoblasts were effectively utilized for individual variant validation using an immunofluorescence assay that we developed.

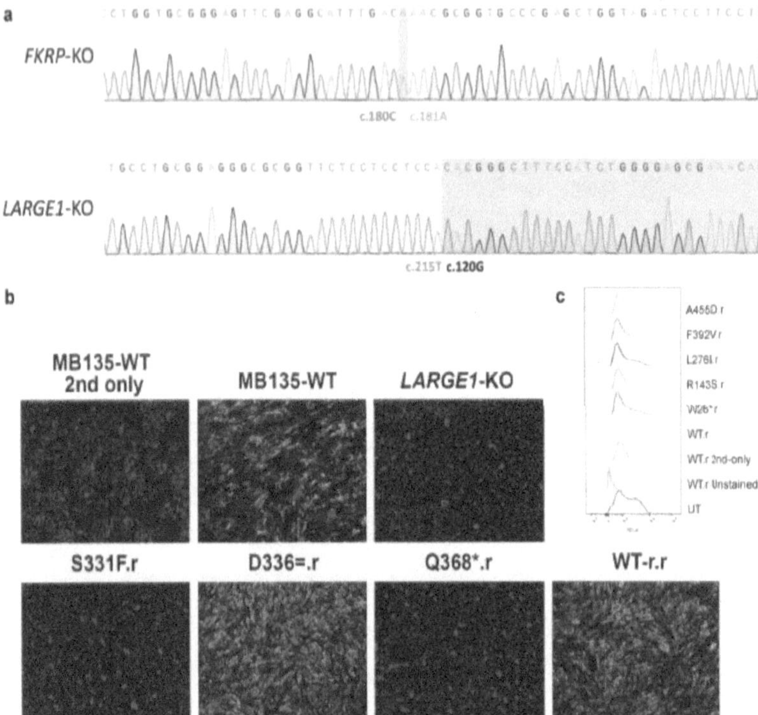

Fig. 2.2.4.1 **Monoclonal homozygous *FKRP*-KO and *LARGE1*-KO MB135 myoblasts were created and individual validations confirmed SMuRF findings in the myogenic context. a,** Homozygous *GOI*-KO MB135 monoclonal cell lines were isolated from pooled CRISPR RNP nucleofected cells. *FKRP*-KO MB135 carries a 1-bp frameshifting insertion (c.181Adup). *LARGE1*-KO MB135 carries a 94-bp frameshifting deletion (c.121_214del). The mutations were validated with Sanger sequencing. These mutations are the same as the mutations in the *GOI*-KO HAP1 lines. **b,** Validation of individual *LARGE1* variants using an IIH6C7 IF assay. ".r" denotes lentiviral transduction of an individual variant. Green: IIH6C4, α-DG the glycosylation level. Four individual transductions were performed, including and 3 variants. The *LARGE1* sequence was cloned from HEK293T cDNA. HEK293T carries a heterozygous *LARGE1* mutation (c.1848G>A, p.Met616Ile). This variant was removed when building the *LARGE1* SMuRF lentiviral pools but were kept in this experiment depicted in this figure. Sanger sequencing confirmed the frequency of this mutation in these four lentiviral constructs were: WT 35.1%, S331F 96.3%, D336= 2.0%, Q368*=2.0%. The brightness and contrast of the photos were adjusted in Adobe Photoshop with the same settings. **c,** MB135 is not compatible with the flow cytometric assay due to high background noise. Monoclonal Lenti-*DAG1 FKRP*-KO MB135 myoblasts were used in this IIH6C4 flow cytometric experiment. High background noise was observed in both the control sample where no Lenti-*FKRP* rescue was performed (UT), and the control sample where the Lenti-*FKRP*-rescued cells were stained with secondary antibody but without the IIH6C4 primary antibody (WT.r 2nd-only). No significant differences were observed among different variants. (Monoclonal *FKRP*-KO MB135 myoblasts were also tested and showed the same pattern).

The *FKRP*-KO and *LARGE1*-KO MB135 myoblasts were rescued by different individual variants using lentivirus and differentiated into myotubes for IIH6C4 IF staining (Fig. 2.2.4.2a and Fig. 2.2.4.1b). The results were consistent with the SMuRF scores, the mini-library screen (Fig. 2.1.2.4a,b) and the ClinVar reports. Again, the founder mutation Leu276Ile displayed an intermediate α-DG glycosylation signal, lying between the benign variants and the other pathogenic variants.

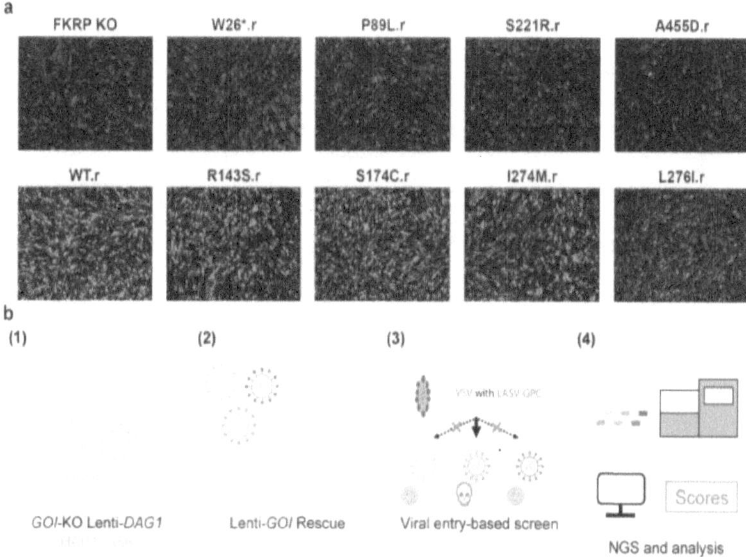

Fig. 2.2.4.2 Validations confirmed SMuRF findings in the myogenic context. a, Validation of individual *FKRP* variants using an IIH6C7 IF assay. The myoblasts underwent transduction and drug selection, followed by differentiation into myotubes, which were subsequently used for IF. ".r" denotes lentiviral transduction of an individual variant. Blue: DAPI. Green: IIH6C4, α-DG the glycosylation level. Nine individual transductions were performed, including WT and 8 variants. The brightness and contrast of the photos were adjusted in Adobe Photoshop with the same settings. **b,** An orthogonal assay based on α-DG-dependent viral entry. Vesicular stomatitis virus (VSV) with Lassa fever virus glycoprotein complex (LASV-GPC) can infect cells in an α-DG-dependent manner. Variant enrichment before/after VSV infection can be used to quantify their performances regarding α-DG glycosylation.

Additionally, we explored an orthogonal assay to further validate SMuRF results. Proper glycosylation of α-DG is crucial for the viral entry of Lassa fever virus (LASV) [218]. LASV glycoprotein complex (LASV-GPC) has been employed to generate recombinant vesicular stomatitis virus (rVSV-LASV-GPC) as a safer agent for investigating LASV entry [219]. rVSV-LASV-GPC was utilized in a gene-trap screen in HAP1 cells to identify crucial genes involved in α-DG glycosylation, where cells with dysfunctional α-DG glycosylation genes exhibited increased resistance to rVSV-LASV-GPC infection, resulting in their enrichment in the population [178].

We adapted this methodology and utilized rVSV-LASV-GPC/ppVSV-LASV-GPC to infect Lenti-*GOI* variant pool-rescued *GOI*-KO MB135 myoblasts (Fig. 2.2.4.2b). The rVSV genome incorporates the LASV-GPC coding sequence, allowing it to re-enter cells. In contrast, the ppVSV lacks this capability as it is pseudotyped using a LASV-GPC plasmid (2.3). Likely due to the re-entering feature of rVSV, the rVSV screen did not yield meaningful results (Fig. 2.2.4.3a). The ppVSV screen for both FKRP and LARGE1 showed a tendency where start-loss variants were the most enriched in the infected group, suggesting a higher disruptive effect on α-DG glycosylation. Nonsense variants were the next most enriched, followed by missense variants, while synonymous variants were the least enriched (Fig. 2.2.4.3b,c). This tendency aligns with what we observed in the SMuRF FACS assay. However, the ppVSV assay, in general, lacks the sensitivity to distinguish differences among the variants.

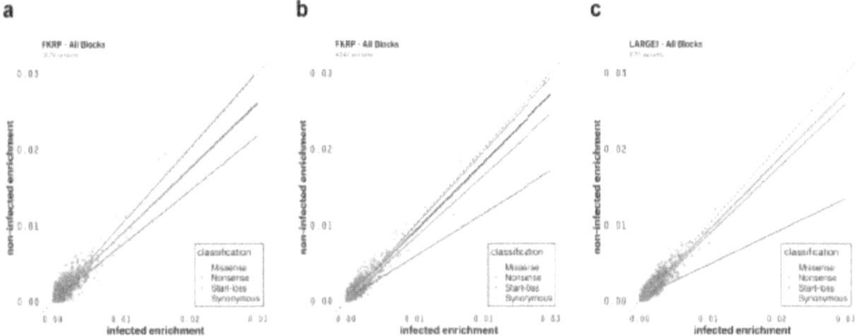

Fig. 2.2.4.3 The VSV-based viral entry assays did not exhibit sufficient sensitivity for large-scale evaluation of variants. Dashed line indicates no enrichment difference between the VSV-infected group and the non-infected group. Black solid line represent linear regression for all variants. Other solid lines represent linear regression for different variant types. **a**, rVSV-LASV-GPC viral entry assay for *FKRP* (The trend lines of missense variants and all variants overlay with the trend line of synonymous variants). ppVSV-LASV-GPC viral entry assay for *FKRP* (**b**) and *LARGE1* (**c**; The trend line of all variants overlay with the trend line of missense variants). The trend lines indicated a tendency where start-loss variants were the most enriched in the infected group, suggesting a greater disruptive effect on α-DG glycosylation. Nonsense variants showed the next highest enrichment, followed by missense variants, while synonymous variants demonstrated the lowest level of enrichment. However, overall, the VSV assays lack sufficient sensitivity for accurate interpretation of variants.

2.2.5 "SMuRFy Secrets": Considerations for the implementation of SMuRF

The lack of definitive diagnoses for rare disease patients is a significant challenge faced in clinical practice. The presence of VUSs in patient genes poses a challenge for clinicians in establishing the disease-causing gene and making informed decisions regarding the suitability of gene-specific treatments. Consequently, such patients are often excluded from receiving appropriate treatments or participating in clinical trials involving novel therapeutics. In this context, the implementation of SMuRF can be beneficial: SMuRF scores can serve as an additional line of evidence to support clinical variant interpretation, aiding in the diagnostic process.

However, in clinical practice, the majority of patients exhibit compound mutations, which raises the need for further investigation on how to apply SMuRF scores in diagnosing such cases. In this study, we employed a naive additive model where the biallelic functional scores were calculated by the simple addition of the SMuRF scores of the variants on both alleles. While this model demonstrated a promising correlation between SMuRF scores and disease severity (Fig. 2.2.2.1c,d), further assessments may be needed. Additionally, our results emphasized the significance of well-curated reports in predicting disease severity (Fig. 2.2.2.3). While our findings revealed a correlation between the disease onset age and SMuRF scores (Fig. 2.2.2.1d and Fig. 2.2.5.1), creatine kinase (CK) values did not show a significant correlation with SMuRF scores (Fig. 2.2.5.2). This observation is consistent with the knowledge in the field that CK levels can fluctuate with activity and decrease when muscle mass is lost over time [220].

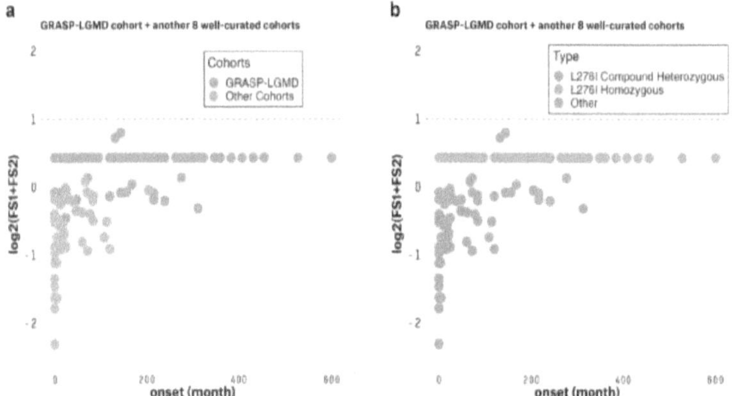

Fig. 2.2.5.1 Variability in onset time among patients with homozygous p.Leu276Ile mutation. Data from The Genetic Resolution and Assessments Solving Phenotypes in LGMD consortium (GRASP LGMD) were integrated with the 8 well-curated cohorts shown in Fig. 2.2.2.1c,d. The GRASP LGMD cohort mainly includes patients with homozygous p.Leu276Ile mutation and patients with compound heterozygous mutations (with p.Leu276Ile on one allele). Patients with homozygous p.Leu276Ile mutation exhibited a diverse range of onset ages, suggesting that the severity of dystroglycanopathy in these individuals might be influenced by other factors in addition to the FKRP mutation. FS1, the functional score of the variant on Allele1; FS2, the functional score of the variant on Allele2. Blue dashed line represents homozygous WT functional score.

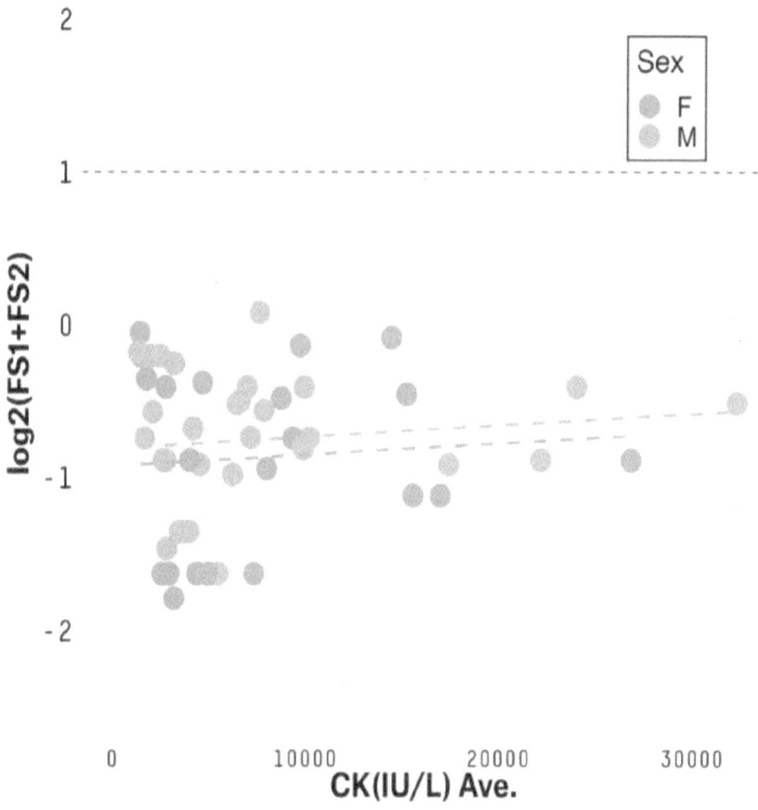

Fig. 2.2.5.2 Creatine kinase (CK) values did not show a significant correlation with SMuRF scores. Patient data were aggregated from 8 published well-curated cohorts. The SMuRF scores are not significantly correlated with the CK values. Spearman's rank correlation rho: -0.05 (all data), 0.03 (male), -0.07 (female). Light grey rectangle indicates the normal range in healthy people (24.00 - 204.00 IU/L). Dashed lines represent linear regression. FS1, the functional score of the variant on Allele1; FS2, the functional score of the variant on Allele2. Blue dashed line represents homozygous WT functional score.

An important consideration in the clinical implementation of the SMuRF score is that the IIH6C4 assay may only capture one of the multiple functions associated with a gene. For example, FKRP is also known to participate in the glycosylation of fibronectin [221]. Hence, a gene variant may have a limited impact on function in the context of a specific assay but may have potentially damaging effects in another assay.

Furthermore, the clinical implementation of the SMuRF score poses challenges in three additional aspects. Firstly, the presence of a homologous gene may impact the clinical relevance of the SMuRF scores. For instance, *LARGE2*, a paralog of *LARGE1* resulting from a duplication event first observed in Chondrichthyes [173], may act as an effective modifier in *LARGE1*-related diseases [222-224]. Secondly, the SMuRF score for nonsense mutations has inherent limitations. In the context of the CDS constructs used in SMuRF, a nonsense mutation does not trigger exon-junction complex (EJC)-enhanced NMD. However, in the correct multi-exon genomic context, when a nonsense mutation is located upstream of the last EJC, it undergoes EJC-dependent NMD, further eliminating any residual functions that the truncated proteins may possess [225]. Lastly, the IIH6C4 assay used in SMuRF may detect technical signals without physiological significance. This is particularly relevant for LARGE1 as LARGE1 is directly involved in the formation of matriglycan, the target of IIH6C4. Specifically, the difference between *LARGE1* missense variants in the GlcAT domain and the XylT domain may be partly technical (Fig. 2.2.3.2c).

SMuRF effectively recapitulated the selection against pathogenic variants by utilizing AF data from gnomAD v3.1.2. Interestingly, we observed a discrepancy between gnomAD v3.1.2 and v2.1.1. Notably, the *FKRP* c.1027G>C(p.Glu343Gln) variant exhibits a 100-fold higher AF in v2 compared to v3, primarily attributed to the limited coverage in the exome data in v2. This again highlights the importance of sequencing larger populations to improve our understanding of variants [226]. A noteworthy aspect of the population study is that the variants favored by selection may not necessarily correspond to the ones that confer optimal enzymatic activity. α-DG glycosylation plays a crucial role in LASV viral entry. It is possible that certain variants, despite conferring lower enzymatic activity for α-DG glycosylation, are favored by selection in populations where LASV is epidemic [209,227].

The lentiviral expression level is essential in the SMuRF workflow. Its significance lies in the fact that for certain variants that compromise the enzymatic activity, the negative impact can be counteracted through the over-expression of the enzyme [181]. This was demonstrated during the early development stage of SMuRF, where we initially attempted to use the EF-1α core promoter to drive the *FKRP* expression and failed to achieve the expected separation (Fig. 2.2.5.3). This aspect is especially relevant in the context of the lentiviral expression system, where the lentiviral expression level can vary from the endogenous level, resulting from the complex effects of both copy numbers and promoter strength.

a

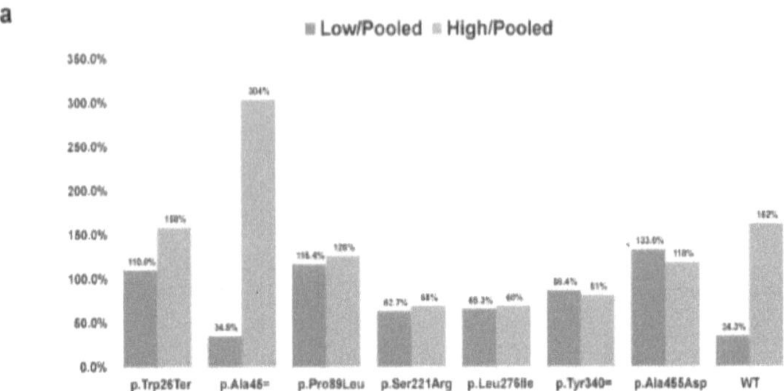

b

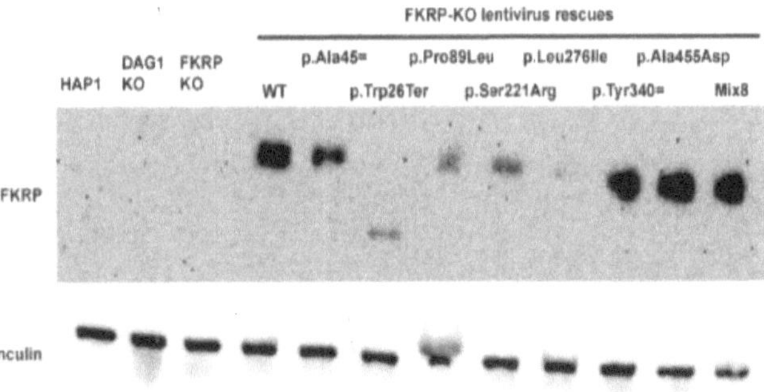

Fig. 2.2.5.3 EF1α-driven over-expression masks pathogenic effects of variants. These results were from experiments in the early development stage. The platform cell line is the *FKRP*-KO cell line without Lenti-*DAG1* transduction. Initially, we constructed Lenti-EF1α-*FKRP*-P2A-BSD, with an EF-1α core promoter driving the expression of a fused protein of FKRP and Blasticidin S deaminase (BSD), linked by a P2A self-cleaving peptide coding sequence. We later abandoned this design as the over-expression failed to generate the expected separation and the fusion impeded our ability to study nonsense variants in an unbiased manner. However, this early design was used in the experiments in this figure. Interestingly, the cells treated with the lentivirus carrying the p.Trp26Ter nonsense mutation unexpectedly survived the blasticidin drug selection, suggesting the existence of a genetic mechanism that could rescue this nonsense mutation, at least in the context of using this construct. **a**, A mini-library comprising 7 *FKRP* variants and the WT sequence was employed in a FACS experiment. The over-expression masked the deleterious effects of the pathogenic variants, leading to a lack of significant enrichment differences of those variants between the high-glycosylation and low-glycosylation populations. (The enrichment was quantified by Sanger sequencing peaks; the enrichment of the WT was calculated based on the enrichments of other variants.) **b**, Western blot was performed for individually transduced samples as well as the Mix8 sample. The lentiviral expression was excessively high compared to the endogenous *FKRP* expression in WT HAP1 (not detectable by WB). A smaller band (between 35 kDa and 55 kDa) was detected in the p.Trp26Ter sample, supporting the hypothesis of the existence of a downstream alternative start codon rescuing this mutation (likely, Met144, resulting in a 39.0 kDa product).

The impact of the Multiplicity of Infection (MOI) of the lentiviral pool on the outcome of the functional characterization is profound (Fig. 2.2.5.4). In the SMuRF workflow, the MOI was controlled to ensure that the lentiviral GOI RNA level is comparable to the endogenous level in WT cells. The titer was determined in pre-experiments. Future improvement to the workflow entails identifying and employing the endogenous promoter core element as a replacement for the UbC promoter [228], or employing saturation mutagenesis methods that can introduce variants to the correct genomic context [229].

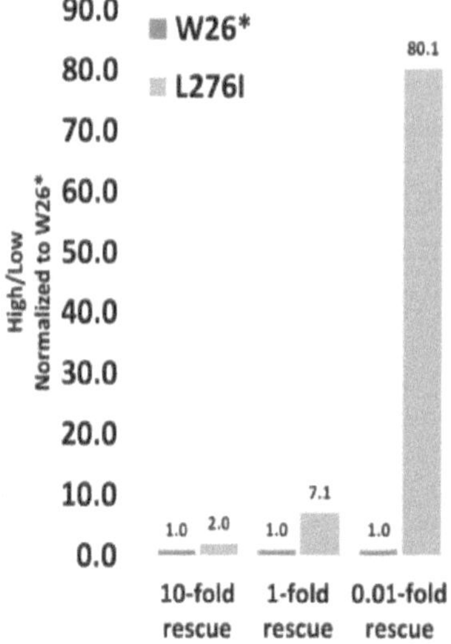

Fig. 2.2.5.4 **The impact of the MOI of the lentiviral pool on the outcome of the functional characterization is profound.** A small-scale FACS experiment utilizing an FKRP mini-library comprising WT, Trp26Ter, and Leu276Ile. y-axis is high/low enrichment normalized to Trp26Ter. Higher number indicates higher function. 1-fold transduction conferred lentiviral *FKRP* expression comparable to the

endogenous *FKRP* expression in WT cells. Higher MOI appeared to reduce the functional difference between Trp26Ter and Leu276Ile.

Synonymous variants are typically considered to have limited effects on gene function [230]. In our study, we adopted the assumption that synonymous variants have no effects when calculating our confidence scores. However, it is possible that some synonymous variants can affect RNA motifs, structure, or splicing, leading to potential changes in gene function [231-233]. While evaluating the effects of variants on splicing is challenging within the current SMuRF framework due to its dependence on CDS-only constructs, it is possible that the effects of synonymous variants on RNA motifs can be captured by SMuRF. Indeed, we identified two synonymous variants in *LARGE1*, c.639T>C (SMuRF=1.18) and c.642A>G (SMuRF score=1.22), which may have gain-of-function effects by removing a poly(A) motif from the coding sequence (Fig. 2.2.5.5). The poly(A) signal is associated with transcription termination, and its removal may increase the level of functional transcripts [234]. However, despite this poly(A) motif is not separated by exon junctions *in vivo*, it is still important to note that this observation may not fully apply to the endogenous *LARGE1* due to regulatory mechanisms unique to the correct genomic context.

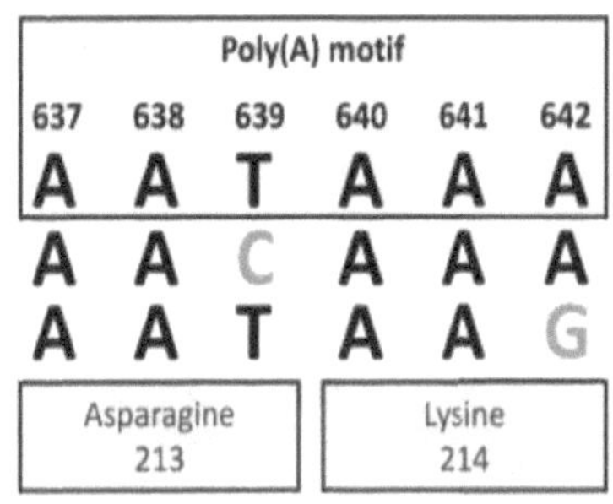

Fig. 2.2.5.5 SMuRF has the potential to capture the effects of synonymous variants on RNA motifs. Two synonymous variants (red) in *LARGE1*, c.639T>C (p.Asn213=) (SMuRF=1.18) and c.642A>G (p.Lys214=) (SMuRF=1.22), may potentially have gain-of-function effects by removing a poly(A) motif from the coding sequence.

One of the motivations to develop SMuRF was to democratize DMS so that modestly funded laboratories that are experts in particular disease genes can contribute to the community effort to achieve an "Atlas of Variant Effects". SMuRF achieved this democratization with inexpensive reagents, commonly used laboratory equipment, and open-source software for data analysis (2.3). SMuRF can be readily adapted for studying other enzymes involved in α-DG glycosylation. In this thesis, we employed SMuRF to analyze all possible coding SNVs of *FKRP* and *LARGE1*, as this type of variant is the most common causal variant observed in dystroglycanopathies. However, it is worth noting that the PALS-C saturation mutagenesis method developed for SMuRF can be applied to small-sized variants beyond SNVs, including SAAS and small insertions or deletions. Moreover, integrating PALS-C with other functional assays specific to other genes or regulatory elements can further enhance the versatility of SMuRF.

2.3 Materials and Methods for SMuRF

Cell culture:

Wildtype HAP1 (C631) and *DAG1*-KO HAP1 (HZGHC000120c016) were ordered from Horizon Discovery. All HAP1 cells were cultured in Iscove's Modified Dulbecco's Medium (IMDM) (Gibco, 12440053) with 10% Fetal Bovine Serum (FBS, R&D Systems, S11150) and 1× Antibiotic-Antimycotic (Anti-anti, Gibco, 15240062). The medium was replaced every 2 days, unless otherwise stated. HAP1 cells tend to grow into multi-layers; hence, to keep the cells in optimal status, TrypLE Express Enzyme (Gibco, 12605010) was used to passage the cells to maintain the cells in healthy confluency (30-90%). The HAP1 cells used in SMuRF were immortalized using lentivirus packaged with pLV-hTERT-IRES-hygro (Addgene, 85140), a gift from Tobias Meyer, as previously described [235]. HEK293T cells were cultured in DMEM (Gibco, 11995065) with 10% FBS and 1× Anti-anti. All MB135 cells were cultured in Ham's F-10 Nutrient Mix (Gibco, 11550043) with 20% FBS, 1× Anti-anti, 51 ng/ml dexamethasone (Sigma-Aldrich, D2915) and 10 ng/mL basic fibroblast growth factor (EMD/Millipore, GF003AF-MG). The medium was replaced every 2 days, unless otherwise stated. The MB135 cells were differentiated in Skeletal Muscle Differentiation Medium (PromoCell, C-23061) with 1× Anti-anti. The differentiation medium was replaced every 4 days, unless otherwise stated.

CRISPR RNP nucleofection:

Synthetic Single Guide RNA (sgRNA) Kits and SpCas9 2NLS Nuclease were ordered from Synthego. RNP complexes were prepared in SE Cell Line Nucleofector

Solution (Lonza, PBC1-00675) and delivered into cells with a Lonza 4D-Nucleofector. The program used for HAP1 was EN-138; the program used for MB135 was CA-137. Single clones were isolated from pooled nucleofected cells and genotyped by targeted Sanger sequencing. *FKRP*-KO HAP1 carries a 1-bp insertion (c.181Adup); *FKRP*-KO MB135 is homozygous for the same mutation. *LARGE1*-KO HAP1 carries a 94-bp deletion (c.121_214del); *LARGE1*-KO MB135 is homozygous for the same mutation.

FKRP-KO sgRNA		GTTCGAGGCATTTGACAACG
LARGE1-KO sgRNAs (used as a mixture)		GATGGGATGGGGCTCGGCCC
		GGTGCGCATGCGCGAGGTGG
		TCCAGCGGTGACAGAGACAC
RNP preparation	18 μL supplemented SE Solution + 6 μL 30 μM sgRNA + 1 μL 20 μM Cas9	
	Room temperature 10 mins	
	Add to 150 k cells (spun down 100 × g, 10 mins; resuspended in 5 μL supplemented SE Solution)	
	SE Cell Line 4D-Nucleofector X Kit S was used (Lonza, V4XC-1032)	
Pick single clones	Allow the nucleofected cells to recover in the growth medium	
	Plate the nucleofected cells sparsely and allow them to form monoclonal clusters	
	Pick monoclonal cells under microscope	
Genotyping primers	FKRP-GT-F	CATCACCCTCAACCTTCTGGTC
	FKRP-GT-R	CATCAGGTACTAGGGCCACAAACTC
	LARGE1-GT-F	GGCAATCGGGACTTTGGACA
	LARGE1-GT-R	GCCTCGCCATGTAGTAAGGG

Table 2.3.1 Generating the *GOI*-KO cell lines.

Plasmid construction:

Lenti-*DAG1* plasmid used the backbone of lentiCRISPR v2, which was a gift from Feng Zhang (Addgene, 52961). *DAG1* coding exons were cloned from human genome DNA by PCR. Lenti-*FKRP* plasmids and Lenti-*LARGE1* plasmids used the backbone of lentiCas9-Blast, which was a gift from Feng Zhang (Addgene, 52962). *FKRP* coding exon was cloned from HAP1 genome DNA. *LARGE1* coding sequence was cloned from HEK293T cDNA. HEK293T carries a *LARGE1* mutation (c.1848G>A) on one allele, which was removed from the Lenti-*LARGE1* plasmids to make the pooled variant library. The removal of this mutation used the same strategy as the introduction of individual variants to the lentiviral plasmids for the mini-libraries: briefly, a short localized region was cut with restriction enzymes from the wildtype plasmid and 2 variant-carrying inserts, each covering 1 of 2 sides of this region were inserted. The UbC promoter was cloned from pAAV-UbC-eGFP-F, which was a gift from Pantelis Tsoulfas (Addgene, 71545). The EF-1α promoter was taken from lentiGuide-Puro, which was a gift from Feng Zhang (Addgene, 52963). BSD-WPRE was from lentiCas9-Blast. The lentiviral plasmids used for the pooled library contain a UbC-driven gene-of-interest CDS and an EF-1α-driven BSD. Plasmid assemblies were achieved either with NEBuilder HiFi DNA Assembly Master Mix (NEB, E2621) or T4 DNA Ligase (M0202).

Q5 High-Fidelity DNA Polymerase (NEB, M0491SVIAL) was used for the PCR reactions according to the manufacturers' manuals.	
Oxford Nanopore long-read sequencing services were provided by Plasmidsaurus to validate the plasmid sequences.	
The *DAG1* CDS sequence in this project	ENST00000308775.7
	but carrying a common variants c.41C>G (p.Ser14Trp)
	The AF of this variant is 0.9762 in gnomAD v3
The *FKRP* CDS sequence in this project	ENST00000318584.10
The *LARGE1* CDS sequence in this project	ENST00000354992.7
Primers for CDS plasmid construction (*The overhangs were designed according to different assembly scheme):	
DAG1-Exon2-F	GGTTCTAGAGCGCTGCCACCATGAGGATGTCTGTGGGCCTC
DAG1-Exon2-R	CCGCTGATACCTTGATGATATCTCCACTGGAGGCAAT
DAG1-Exon3-F	TATCATCAAGGTATCAGCGGCAGGGAAGGAG
DAG1-Exon3-R	AAGTTTGTTGCGCCGGATCCAGGTGGGACATAGGGAGGAGG
FKRP-clone-F (matching part*)	ATGCGGCTCACCCGCT
FKRP-clone-R (matching part*)	GCCGCTTCCCGTCAGA
LARGE1-clone-F (matching part*)	ATGCTGGGAATCTGCAGGG
LARGE1-clone-R (matching part*)	CTAGCTGTTGTTCTCGGCTGTGAG
UbC-clone-F (matching part*)	GGCCTCCGCGCCGG
UbC-clone-R (matching part*)	ACCAAGTGACGATCACAGCGATCC
EF1α-clone-F (matching part*)	GGCTCCGGTGCCCGTCA
EF1α-clone-R (matching part*)	GGTGGCCGTACGTCACGACA
BSD-WPRE-clone-F (matching part*)	ATGGCCAAGCCTTTGTCTCAAGAAG

BSD-WPRE-clone-R (matching part*)	GCGGGGAGGCGGCC
Two cloning strategies to introduce individual variant to the WT plasmid:	
Cut and Swap: A short localized region was cut with restriction enzymes from the wildtype plasmid to serve as the backbone. Two variant-carrying inserts were amplified using PCR. The variant of interest was introduced in the R primer for the 5' insert and the F primer for the 3' insert. The backbone and those two inserts were assembled with NEBuilder HiFi DNA Assembly Master Mix (NEB, E2621)	
Site-directed mutagenesis: The whole plasmid was amplified using a pair of primers carrying the variant of interest. The WT plasmid was removed from the reaction using Type2M enzyme DpnI (NEB, R0176S). F primers were designed as: (5'->3') 7-bp flanking sequence A + 1-bp variant + 7-bp flanking sequence B + 15-bp matching sequence; R primers were designed as (5'->3') 7-bp flanking sequence B + 1-bp variant + 7-bp flanking sequence A + 15-bp matching sequence.	
Plasmids deposited to Addgene:	
Lenti-*DAG1*	205149
Lenti-UbC-*FKRP*-EF1α-*BSD*	205150
Lenti-UbC-*LARGE1*-EF1α-*BSD*	205151

Table 2.3.2 Cloning details of plasmid construction and the list of plasmids deposited to Addgene.

RT-PCR and RT-qPCR:

RT-PCR and RT-qPCR were performed following manufacturers' manuals. PrimeScript RT Reagent Kit (Takara, RR037) was used for cDNA synthesis. Phusion High-Fidelity DNA Polymerase (NEB, M0530) was used for PCR reactions. SsoAdvanced Universal SYBR Green Supermix (Bio-Rad, 1725271), Hard-Shell 96-Well PCR Plates (Bio-Rad, HSP9601), Plate Sealing Film (Bio-Rad, MSB1001) and Bio-Rad C1000 Touch Thermal Cycler were used for qPCR experiments.

DAG1-cDNA-F	GATCTGCTACCGCAAGAAGC
DAG1-cDNA-R	ATGGTGTCCTGGTTCAGAGG
FKRP-rtPCR-F	TGGGCATCTACTTGGAGGAC
FKRP-rtPCR-R	TTGCTTTCGCTGTACTGCAC
LARGE1-cDNA-F	GAGCAGTGCTACAGAGACGTGT
LARGE1-cDNA-R	TGCCGTCATACTCCAGGAAGGT
LARGE1-gDNA-F	ATCAGCCTGGCCCTCTACC
LARGE1-gDNA-R	TGTAGGGAGTGCTGATGTGC

Table 2.3.3 RT-(q)PCR and qPCR primers used in the development of SMuRF.

Lentivirus packaging and transduction:

Lentivirus was packaged by HEK293T cells. For a 10-cm dish (90% confluency), 1.5 mL Opti-MEM (Gibco, 31985062), 10 μg psPAX2 (Addgene, 12260), 2 μg pMD2.G (Addgene, 12259), 9 μg lentiviral plasmid, and 50 μL TransIT-LT1 Transfection Reagent (Mirus, MIR 2300) were mixed at room temperature for 15 mins and then added to the cells. 3.5 mL DMEM was added to the cells. 72 hrs later, the supernatant in the dish was filtered with 0.45 μm PES filter (Thermo Scientific, 165-0045), mixed with 5 mL Lenti-X Concentrator (Takara, 631232) and rocked at 4 °C overnight. The viral particles were then spun down (1800 ×g, 4 °C, 1hr) and resuspended in 200 μL DMEM. Lentivirus was titrated with Lenti-X GoStix Plus (Takara, 631280). For lentiviral transduction, the cells to be transduced were plated in wells of plates. One day after seeding, the medium was replaced and suppled with polybrene (final conc. 8 μg/mL). Lentivirus was then added to the wells for a spinfection (800 ×g, 30 °C, 1hr). One day post-transduction, the medium was replaced, and drug selection was started if applicable. For constructs with BSD, Blasticidin S HCl (Gibco, A1113903, final conc. 5 μg/mL) was used for drug selection. For constructs with PuroR, Puromycin Dihydrochloride (Gibco, A1113803, final conc. 1 μg/mL) was used. Drug selection was performed for 10-14 days.

<u>PALS-C cloning for saturation mutagenesis:</u>

Each variant of all possible CDS SNVs (Fig. 2.1.2.3a,b) was included in a 64-bp ssDNA oligo. The oligos were synthesized (one pool per GOI) by Twist Bioscience. PALS-C is an 8-step cloning strategy to clone lentiviral plasmid pools from the oligos. An elaborate protocol can be found in Table 2.3.4. Briefly, the oligos were used as PCR reverse primers, which were annealed to the plasmid template and extended towards the 5' end of the gene of interest. The resulting products of each block were isolated using block-specific primers. Then the variant strands were extended towards the 3' end to get the full-length sequences, which were subsequently inserted into the plasmid backbone using NEBuilder (NEB, E2621). The purifications for PALS-C steps were done with NucleoSpin Gel and PCR Clean-Up kit (Takara, 740609). Final assembled products were delivered to Endura Electrocompetent Cells (Lucigen, 60242-1) via electrotransformation (Bio-Rad Gene Pulser II). Transformed bacteria were grown overnight and plasmid pools were extracted using the PureLink Midiprep Kit (Invitrogen, K210014).

Primers used for PALS-C:			
PALS-C-universal-F1	GAACAGGCGAGGAAAAGTAG		
PALS-C-universal-F2	GATCGTCACTTGGTACCGGTTCTAGA		
PALS-C-universal-R2-FKRP	TGGCACTTTTCGGGGGATCCTC		
PALS-C-universal-R2-LARGE1	TGGCACTTTTCGGGGGATCCCT		
Plasmid templates:			
Lenti-UbC-FKRP-EF1α-BSD			
Lenti-UbC-LARGE1-EF1α-BSD			
R1 oligos were generated using the following python scripts (github.com/leklab/Balthazar):			
PALS_C_oligos_FKRP.py			
PALS_C_oligos_LARGE1.py			
R1 oligo structure (5'->3'):			
1	8-nt block specific adaptor		
2	Type2S enzyme recognition site		
3	5-nt block specific insulator (the 3' 4-nt sequence does not appear in this block)		
4	19-nt GOI downstream sequence		
5	Variant		
6	25-nt GOI upstream sequence		
Reagents:			
1	Q5 Reaction Buffer (NEB, B9027SVIAL)	7	BsmBI-v2 (NEB, R0739S)
2	Q5 High GC Enhancer (NEB, B9028AVIAL)	8	BsaI-HFv2 (NEB, R3733S)
3	10 mM dNTPs (NEB, N0447)	9	DpnI (NEB, R0176S)
4	Q5 High-Fidelity DNA Polymerase (NEB, M0491SVIAL)	10	MspJI (NEB, R0661S)
5	NEBuilder HiFi DNA Assembly Master Mix (NEB, E2621)	11	XbaI (NEB, R0145S)

6	Endura Electrocompetent Cells (Lucigen, 60242)		12	BamHI-HF (NEB, R3136S)
PALS-C Step1:				
Q5 Rxn buffer	10 μL	Reaction conditions (*decided based on the product that is the most difficult to amplify):		
Q5 Enh buffer	10 μL			
10 mM dNTPs	1 μL	1	98 °C	hot start
Oligo library (1e6 coverage)	n mol	2	98 °C	4 mins
Plasmid template	n mol	3	Annealing temperature*	20 s
Q5 polymerase	2 μL	4	72 °C	Elongation time*
Water	To 50 μL	5	12 °C	forever
PCR purification with NucleoSpin Gel and PCR Clean-Up Kit (Takara, 740609).				
PALS-C Step2:				
Starting from Step2, the reactions are done independently for different blocks.				
* The input should be decided based on the position of the block. The more distant a block is from the 5' side, the more input is required. Evenly distributed input for all 6 blocks of FKRP generated enough yield for subsequent steps, while the 3' side blocks of LARGE1 required extra input. Step1-2 should be repeated if product yield is insufficient for subsequent steps.				
Q5 Rxn buffer	10 μL	1	98 °C	hot start
Q5 Enh buffer	10 μL	2	98 °C	3 mins
10 mM dNTPs	1 μL	3	98 °C	8 s
Purified Step1 product	*	4	Annealing temperature	20 s
10 μM Universal F1	2.5 μL	5	72 °C	Elongation time
10 μM Block specific R1	2.5 μL	6	Repeat 3-5 for 34 more cycles	
Q5 polymerase	0.5 μL	7	72 °C	5 mins
Water	To 50 μL	8	12 °C	Forever
PCR purification with NucleoSpin Gel and PCR Clean-Up Kit (Takara, 740609).				
PALS-C Step3:				
*BsmBI was used for *FKRP* and BsaI was used for *LARGE1*. The type2S enzymes were picked to avoid the presence of their recognition sites within the CDS.				
Type2S enzyme*	2 μL	Reaction conditions:		
Purified Step2 product	1.2 μg			
Reaction buffer	5 μL	1	Reaction temperature (Lid: 60 °C)	50 mins
Water	To 50 μL	2	12 °C	Forever
Electrophoresis in 1% agarose gel was performed and the bands within the correct size range were cut from the gel; gel purification with NucleoSpin Gel and PCR Clean-Up Kit (Takara, 740609).				
PALS-C Step4:				
purified step3 product + plasmid template = 1000 ng				
purified step3:plasmid template= 1:1 (molar)				
The elongation time should be sufficient for the shortest strand to be elongated to the R2 primer site.				
Q5 Rxn buffer	10 μL	Reaction conditions:		
Q5 Enh buffer	10 μL	1	98 °C	hot start
10 mM dNTPs	1 μL	2	98 °C	5 mins
Purified Step3 product	n mol	3 (optional)	72 °C	5 s
Plasmid template	n mol	4 (optional)	66 °C	20 s
Q5 polymerase*	2 μL	5	72 °C	Elongation time
Water	To 50 μL	6	12 °C	forever
PCR purification with NucleoSpin Gel and PCR Clean-Up Kit (Takara, 740609).				
PALS-C Step5:				
DpnI	0.5 μL	Reaction conditions:		
MspJI	0.5 μL			
CutSmart	5 μL			
Enzyme activator	1 μL			
Purified Step4 product	500 ng	1	37 °C (Lid: 60 °C)	1 hr

Water	To 50 μL	2	12 °C	Forever
Column purification with NucleoSpin Gel and PCR Clean-Up Kit (Takara, 740609). (Follow the PCR purification protocol.)				
PALS-C Step6:				
Q5 Rxn buffer	10 μL	1	98 °C	hot start
Q5 Enh buffer	10 μL	2	98 °C	5 mins
10 mM dNTPs	1.5 μL	3	98 °C	6 s
Purified Step5 product	100 ng	4	Annealing temperature	20 s
10 μM F2	2.5 μL	5	72 °C	Elongation time
10 μM R2	2.5 μL	6	Repeat 3-5 for 34 more cycles	
Q5 polymerase	1 μL	7	72 °C	5 mins
Water	To 50 μL	8	12 °C	Forever
Electrophoresis in 1% agarose gel was performed and the bands with the correct size were cut from the gel; gel purification with NucleoSpin Gel and PCR Clean-Up Kit (Takara, 740609).				
Important: Use 20 μL water or less to dissolve after gel purification; or use a vacuum concentrator to evaporate excess water.				
PALS-C Step7.1:				
XbaI	1.5 μL	Reaction conditions:		
BamHI-HF	1.5 μL			
Plasmid template	3 μg			
CutSmart	5 μL	1	37 °C (Lid: 60 °C)	40 mins
Water	To 50 μL	2	12 °C	Forever
Electrophoresis in 1% agarose gel was performed and the band with the correct size was cut from the gel; gel purification with NucleoSpin Gel and PCR Clean-Up Kit (Takara, 740609).				
PALS-C Step7.2:				
NEBuilderMaster Mix	20 μL	Reaction conditions:		
Backbone	210 ng			
Purified Step6 product	140 ng	1	50 °C (Lid: 60 °C)	60 mins
Water	To 30 μL	2	12 °C	Forever
PALS-C Step8 (for each block):				
Electrocompetent cells	40 μL			
Assembly reaction	4 μL			
Water	160 μL			
1	Split the mixed sample to two pre-chilled 0.1 cm cuvettes (Bio-Rad, 1652089).			
2	Use Bio-Rad Gene Pulser II: (ATTENTION: avoid bubbles) 25 μF; 200 Ohms; 1800 volts.			
3	Add the sample to 900 μL recovery media per cuvette: 250 rpm, 1hr, 37°C.			
4	Combine transformed bacteria from 2 cuvettes.			
5	Add 1/500 volume of the bacteria to 200 μL LB broth and plate it on an ampicillin LB agar plate for quick estimation of complexity.			
	coverage=500*(colony number)/(variant number of a block)			
6	Seed the bacteria in 150 mL LB broth supplemented with ampicillin (100 μg/ml) for overnight culture.			

Table 2.3.4 PALS-C protocol.

To check library complexity, colony forming units (CFUs) were calculated and a minimum 18 × coverage was achieved for the plasmid pool of each block of *FKRP* and

LARGE1. Variants that created new type2S enzyme recognition sites tended to be underrepresented in the pool. These variants are reported here below.

FKRP:					
site	codon	WT_nt	Variant_nt	classification	alert_group
69	23	T	C	Synonymous	group_2
628	210	C	G	Missense	group_2
6	2	G	T	Synonymous	group_2
1034	345	G	T	Missense	group_2
1151	384	G	T	Missense	group_2
145	49	G	C	Missense	group_2
303	101	G	C	Synonymous	group_2
465	155	G	C	Synonymous	group_2
573	191	C	A	Nonsense	group_1
781	261	G	A	Missense	group_1
252	84	C	G	Missense	group_1
909	303	C	G	Missense	group_1
1290	430	C	G	Missense	group_1
439	147	G	A	Missense	group_1
591	197	T	C	Synonymous	group_1
1187	396	A	C	Missense	group_1
357	119	C	G	Synonymous	group_1
879	293	C	G	Synonymous	group_1
975	325	C	G	Synonymous	group_1
LARGE1:					
site	codon	WT_nt	Variant_nt	classification	alert_group
119	40	T	G	Missense	group_2
2176	726	T	G	Missense	group_2
982	328	C	G	Missense	group_2
167	56	C	T	Missense	group_2
1556	519	G	T	Missense	group_2
1713	571	G	T	Synonymous	group_2
1432	478	G	T	Missense	group_2
666	222	G	C	Synonymous	group_2
298	100	A	G	Missense	group_1
559	187	C	G	Missense	group_1
1082	361	C	G	Nonsense	group_1
1859	620	G	A	Missense	group_1
838	280	A	G	Missense	group_1
139	47	T	A	Missense	group_1
269	90	C	A	Missense	group_1
1468	490	G	A	Missense	group_1
1528	510	G	A	Missense	group_1
1963	655	G	A	Missense	group_1
191	64	G	C	Missense	group_1
227	76	A	C	Missense	group_1
338	113	A	C	Missense	group_1

815	272	A	C	Missense	group_1
1347	449	G	C	Missense	group_1
2261	754	A	C	Missense	group_1
26	9	G	C	Missense	group_1
331	111	A	C	Missense	group_1
411	137	A	C	Synonymous	group_1
1117	373	G	C	Missense	group_1
1797	599	A	C	Synonymous	group_1
1994	665	G	C	Missense	group_1

Table 2.3.5 Underrepresented variants due to the limitation of PALS-C. Group1 variants introduce a cut before the variants which will remove the variant from the top strand; Group2 variants introduce a cut after the variants which might affect the elongation of the top strand.

Quality control (QC) of plasmid pools and saturation mutagenesis:

QC was performed for the plasmid pools using the Amplicon-EZ service provided by GENEWIZ (Fig. 2.1.2.3c,d and Table 2.3.6). 99.6% of the SNVs of both genes were represented in the plasmid pools (Fig. 2.1.2.3e,f). Lentivirus of each block was packaged by HEK293T cells in one 10-cm dish. Small-scale pre-experiments were performed to determine the viral dosage for optimal separation. GoStix Value (GV) quantified by the Lenti-X GoStix App (Takara) was used to scale the dosage of each block to be the same. GV is subject to viral-packaging batch effects; hence, lentiviral pools of all blocks were packaged at the same time using the reagents and helper plasmids of the same batch. Depending on the specific batch, 1e3-1e4 GV×μL of lentivirus was used for each block. For each block, 600k HAP1 cells or 200k MB135 cells were plated in a well of a 6-well plate for transduction. The cell number was counted with an Automated Cell Counter (Bio-Rad, TC20). The cell number for each block was expanded to more than 30M for FACS.

Primers used for plasmid pool QC:	
FKRP-QC-block1-F	gccagaacacaggaccggttctaga
FKRP-QC-block1-R	gccaggggcgggtaggggagcgtgt

FKRP-QC-block2-F	gcccagcccgtggtggtggcagccg
FKRP-QC-block2-R	caggctgacgttcagggccaggcac
FKRP-QC-block3-F	cggttgccacggccaaccctgccag
FKRP-QC-block3-R	gctcagccttccagcgcgcgtgggc
FKRP-QC-block4-F	ggcgcgccagcccccgctggccacg
FKRP-QC-block4-R	agccagtagcgcacgcccgcagcct
FKRP-QC-block5-F	gcccgctatgtggtgggcgtgctgg
FKRP-QC-block5-R	gccattgcgggggtagaagggccac
FKRP-QC-block6-F	aaagcaaccacttgcacgtggacct
FKRP-QC-block6-R	gagagaagtttgttgcgccggatcc
LARGE1-NGS-blk1-QC-F	ccctacacgacgctcttccgatctcctacgtcacttggtaccggttctaga
LARGE1-NGS-blk2-QC-F	ccctacacgacgctcttccgatctcctacgtcgcgaggtggaggaggagaa
LARGE1-NGS-blk3-QC-F	ccctacacgacgctcttccgatctcctacgtcggatacaatgccagccggg
LARGE1-NGS-blk4-QC-F	ccctacacgacgctcttccgatctcctacgtgtctgatgaagcttgtcctg
LARGE1-NGS-blk5-QC-F	ccctacacgacgctcttccgatctcctacgtacaggggtgatcctgttact
LARGE1-NGS-blk6-QC-F	ccctacacgacgctcttccgatctcctacgtcgtgtctgatctaaaggtca
LARGE1-NGS-blk7-QC-F	ccctacacgacgctcttccgatctcctacgtgagagcgcttcactgtccac
LARGE1-NGS-blk8-QC-F	ccctacacgacgctcttccgatctcctacgtatgagccgccacaacgtggg
LARGE1-NGS-blk9-QC-F	ccctacacgacgctcttccgatctcctacgtactgcgctaccggctgtcct
LARGE1-NGS-blk10-QC-F	ccctacacgacgctcttccgatctcctacgttaggctttggctggaacaaa
LARGE1-NGS-blk1-QC-R	gactggagttcagacgtgtgctcttccgatctgctgcctgcggagggcgcgg
LARGE1-NGS-blk2-QC-R	gactggagttcagacgtgtgctcttccgatcttttgaccagggtgacgacat
LARGE1-NGS-blk3-QC-R	gactggagttcagacgtgtgctcttccgatctttggcaggaagagtcttggt
LARGE1-NGS-blk4-QC-R	gactggagttcagacgtgtgctcttccgatcttcttccgcagcttatccaga
LARGE1-NGS-blk5-QC-R	gactggagttcagacgtgtgctcttccgatctcttgggggagttccagtgaa
LARGE1-NGS-blk6-QC-R	gactggagttcagacgtgtgctcttccgatctaggaagtacaggtgggtgcg
LARGE1-NGS-blk7-QC-R	gactggagttcagacgtgtgctcttccgatctccttgtacacgatgtggtag
LARGE1-NGS-blk8-QC-R	gactggagttcagacgtgtgctcttccgatctctccgcttttgacttgggga
LARGE1-NGS-blk9-QC-R	gactggagttcagacgtgtgctcttccgatctagctccatgatatgagccac
LARGE1-NGS-blk10-QC-R	gactggagttcagacgtgtgctcttccgatctcacttttcgggggatcccta
NGS-PCR3-F	aatgatacggcgaccaccgagatctacactctttccctacacgacgctcttccgatct
NGS-PCR3-R	caagcagaagacggcatacgagatcgcgcggtgtgactggagttcagacgtgtgctctt

For *FKRP* plasmid pool QC (for the plasmid pool of each block):

Q5 Rxn buffer	10 μL	1	98 °C	hot start
Q5 Enh buffer	10 μL	2	98 °C	3 mins
10 mM dNTPs	1 μL	3	98 °C	6 s
Plasmid	~300 ng	4	70 °C	15 s
10 μM F primer	2.5 μL	5	72 °C	5 s
10 μM R primer	2.5 μL	6	Repeat 3-5 for 32 more cycles	
Q5 polymerase	0.5 μL	7	72 °C	5 mins
Water	To 50 μL	8	12 °C	Forever

Electrophoresis and gel purification (Takara, 740609) were performed.

The purified products were sent for Amplicon-EZ sequencing.

For *LARGE1* plasmid pool QC (for the plasmid pool of each block):

Q5 Rxn buffer	10 μL	1	98 °C	hot start
Q5 Enh buffer	10 μL	2	98 °C	3 mins
10 mM dNTPs	1 μL	3	98 °C	6 s
Plasmid	~50 ng	4	Annealing temperature	15 s
10 μM F primer	2.5 μL	5	72 °C	7 s
10 μM R primer	2.5 μL	6	Repeat 3-5 for 33 more cycles	
Q5 polymerase	0.5 μL	7	72 °C	5 mins

Water	To 50 µL	8	12 °C	Forever
Electrophoresis and gel purification (Takara, 740609) were performed.			Annealing temperature for different blocks	
			61 °C	1, 4, 6, 7
			64 °C	5, 9, 10
			66 °C	2, 3, 8
The purified products were mixed for the following reaction:				
Q5 Rxn buffer	10 µL	1	98 °C	hot start
Q5 Enh buffer	10 µL	2	98 °C	3 mins
10 mM dNTPs	1 µL	3	98 °C	6 s
Mixed purified products	100 ng	4	72 °C	15 s
10 µM NGS-PCR3-F	2.5 µL	5	72 °C	8 s
10 µM NGS-PCR3-R	2.5 µL	6	Repeat 3-5 for 19 more cycles	
Q5 polymerase	1 µL	7	72 °C	5 mins
Water	To 50 µL	8	12 °C	Forever
PCR purification (Takara, 740609) was performed and the sample was sent for Amplicon-EZ sequencing.				
Scripts for the plasmid pool QC analytical pipelines (github.com/leklab/Balthazar):				
FKRP plasmid QC package				
LARGE1 plasmid QC package				

Table 2.3.6 Quality control (QC) of plasmid pools.

Proof-of-concept mini-libraries:

Mini-libraries of variants were employed to examine and optimize the separation of the FACS assay. Lentiviral constructs were cloned and packaged individually for 8 *FKRP* variants and 3 *LARGE1* variants in addition to the wildtype constructs. These lentiviral particles were mixed to make a mix-9 *FKRP* mini-library and a mix-4 *LARGE1* mini-library. Conditions of transduction, staining, sorting and gDNA extraction were optimized using the mini-libraries. Relative enrichment of variants was defined as the ratio of the variants' representation in the high-glycosylation sample to their representation in the low-glycosylation group, which was quantified with either Sanger sequencing or Amplicon-EZ NGS (Table 2.3.7).

Variants in the mini-libraries/used for individual validation:	
Variant	Clinical significance (ClinVar)
NM_024301.5(FKRP):c.77G>A (p.Trp26Ter)	Pathogenic/Likely pathogenic
NM_024301.5(FKRP):c.266C>T (p.Pro89Leu)	Pathogenic/Likely pathogenic
NM_024301.5(FKRP):c.427C>A (p.Arg143Ser)	Benign/Likely benign

NM_024301.5(FKRP):c.520A>T (p.Ser174Cys)		Benign/Likely benign
NM_024301.5(FKRP):c.663C>A (p.Ser221Arg)		Pathogenic
NM_024301.5(FKRP):c.822C>G (p.Ile274Met)		Conflicting interpretations of pathogenicity
NM_024301.5(FKRP):c.826C>A (p.Leu276Ile)		Pathogenic/Likely pathogenic
NM_024301.5(FKRP):c.1364C>A (p.Ala455Asp)		Pathogenic
NM_133642.5(LARGE1):c.992C>T (p.Ser331Phe)		Pathogenic
NM_133642.5(LARGE1):c.1008T>C (p.Asp336=)		Benign
NM_133642.5(LARGE1):c.1102C>T (p.Gln368Ter)		Pathogenic
Primers used for lentiviral sequence isolation:		
PALS-C-universal-F2		gatcgtcacttggtaccggttctaga
PALS-C-universal-R2-FKRP		tggcacttttcgggggatcctc
PALS-C-universal-R2-LARGE1		tggcacttttcgggggatccct
Primers used for *FKRP* Sanger sequencing:		
FKRP-QC-block2-F		gcccagcccgtggtggtggcagccg
FKRP-QC-block3-F		cggttgccacggccaaccctgccag
FKRP-QC-block5-F		gcccgctatgtggtgggcgtgctgg
FKRP-GT-R		catcaggtactagggccacaaactc
Primers used for *FKRP* Amplicon-EZ sequencing:		
Amplicon1	PALS-C-universal-F2	gatcgtcacttggtaccggttctaga
	FKRP-GT-R	catcaggtactagggccacaaactc
Amplicon2	FKRP-QC-block2-F	gcccagcccgtggtggtggcagccg
	FKRP-QC-block3-R	gctcagccttccagcgcgcgtgggc
Amplicon3	FKRP-QC-block3-F	cggttgccacggccaaccctgccag
	FKRP-QC-block3-R	gctcagccttccagcgcgcgtgggc
Amplicon4	FKRP-QC-block4-F	ggcgcgccagcccccgctggccacg
	FKRP-QC-block4-R	agccagtagcgcacgcccgcagcct
Amplicon5	FKRP-QC-block6-F	aaagcaaccacttgcacgtggacct
	FKRP-CDS-backbone-junction-R	gtggcacttttcgggggatcctcagccgcttcccgtcagactc
Primers used for *LARGE1* Sanger sequencing:		
LARGE1-block4-seq-F		ttatggtctgatgaagcttgtcctg

Table 2.3.7 Proof-of-concept mini-libraries and associated primers.

Staining for FFC and FACS:

Reagent volumes were determined based on sample size. Below, the staining for samples of one gene block is described as an example. The cells were washed twice with DPBS (Gibco, 14190144), digested with Versene (Gibco, 15040066), and counted. 30M cells were used for staining, which was performed in a 15 mL tube. The cells were spun down (700 ×g, 4 °C, 15 mins) and resuspended in 3mL DPBS supplemented with 30 μL Viobility 405/452 Fixable Dye (Miltenyi Biotec, 130-130-420). All the following steps were done in the dark. The sample was gently rocked at room temperature for 30 mins, and then 7 mL PEB buffer (1 volume of MACS BSA Stock Solution, Miltenyi Biotec, 130-091-376 ;19 volumes of autoMACS Rinsing Solution, Miltenyi Biotec, 130-091-222) was added to the tube. The cells were spun down (700 ×g, 4 °C, 15 mins) and resuspended in 3mL DPBS supplemented with 30 μL Human BD Fc Block (BD Pharmingen, 564220). The sample was gently rocked at room temperature for 30 mins, and then 7 mL DPBS was added. The cells were spun down (700 ×g, 4 °C, 10 mins) and resuspended in 3mL MAGIC buffer (5% FBS; 0.1% NaAz w/v; 10% 10× DPBS, Gibco, 14200166; water, Invitrogen, 10977015) supplemented with 15 μL IIH6C4 antibody (Sigma-Aldrich, 05-593, discontinued; or antibody made in Dr. Kevin Campbell's lab). The sample was gently rocked at 4 °C for 20 hrs. 7 mL MAGIC buffer was added before the cells were spun down (700 ×g, 4 °C, 10 mins) and resuspended in 3 mL MAGIC buffer supplemented with 60 μL Rabbit anti-Mouse IgM FITC Secondary Antibody (Invitrogen, 31557). The sample was gently rocked at 4 °C for 20 hrs. 7 mL DPBS was added to the sample before the cells were spun down (700 ×g, 4 °C, 10 mins), resuspended with 4 mL DPBS and filtered with 40 μm Cell Strainer (Falcon, 352340). Important: DO NOT use IIH6C4 antibody from Santa Cruz, sc-73586.

FFC and FACS gating parameters:

FFC experiments were performed with a BD LSR II Flow Cytometer; FACS experiments were performed with a BD FACSAria Flow Cytometer. Forward scatter (FSC) and side scatter (SSC) were used to exclude cell debris and multiplets. Singlets were isolated for downstream analysis. Pacific Blue (450/50 BP) or an equivalent channel was used to detect the Viobility 405/452 Fixable Dye and isolate the live cells for analysis. FITC (530/30 BP), GFP (510/20 BP) or an equivalent channel was used to detect the FITC secondary antibody signal. 20k events were recorded for each block to decide the gating parameters. For FACS, the top ~20% of the cells were isolated as the high-glycosylation group and the bottom ~40% of the cells were isolated as the low-glycosylation group. The .fcs files, the FlowJo .wsp files and the software interface reports of the sorter were made available on FlowRepository. A minimum ~1000 × coverage (*e.g.*, 750k cells harvested for a block with 750 variants) was achieved for both groups of each block.

NGS library construction:

The cells were spun down (800 ×g, 4 °C, 10 mins), and gDNA was harvested from each sample with PureLink Genomic DNA Mini Kit (Invitrogen, K182002). A 3-step PCR library construction was performed to build the sequencing library. Step1: lentiviral sequence isolation. A pair of primers specific to the lentiviral backbone was used to amplify the lentiviral CDS sequences of each sample. Step2: block isolation. Each primer contained a 20-bp flanking sequence of the specific block and a partial Illumina adaptor sequence. F primers contained the barcodes to distinguish the high-glycosylation group and the low-glycosylation group. Step3: adaptor addition. Step2 products were multiplexed and the rest of the Illumina adaptor was added to the amplicons. An elaborate protocol can be found in Table 2.3.8. The NGS libraries were sequenced using Psomagen's HiSeq X service. ~400M reads were acquired per library.

PCR1:	
PCR1-F	GATCGTCACTTGGTACCGGTTCTAGA
PCR1-R (FKRP)	TGGCACTTTTCGGGGGATCCTC
PCR1-R (LARGE1)	TGGCACTTTTCGGGGGATCCCT

Reaction conditions:				
Q5 Reaction Buffer	10 μL	Step1	98 °C	Hot start
Q5 High GC Enhancer	10 μL	Step2	98 °C	3 mins
10 mM dNTPs	1 μL	Step3	98 °C	8 s
Q5 High-Fidelity DNA Polymerase	1 μL	Step4	68 °C	20 s
10μM PCR1-F	2.5 μL	Step5	72 °C	45 s
10μM PCR1-R	2.5 μL	Step 3-5, 35 cycles		
gDNA	0.3-1 μg	Step6	72 °C	5 mins
Nuclease-Free Water	To 50 μL	Step7	12 °C	Infinite

Electrophoresis in 1% agarose gel. Product band size is 1534 bp (FKRP) or 2317 bp (LARGE1). Gel purification with NucleoSpin Gel and PCR Clean-Up Kit (Takara, 740609). Elute with 25 μL Nuclease-Free Water.

PCR2:	
FKRP-blk1-high-F	ccctacacgacgctcttccgatcttacacgatccacttggtaccggttctaga
FKRP-blk2-high-F	ccctacacgacgctcttccgatcttacacgatcgcccgtggtggtggcagccg
FKRP-blk3-high-F	ccctacacgacgctcttccgatcttacacgatcgccacggccaaccctgccag
FKRP-blk4-high-F	ccctacacgacgctcttccgatcttacacgatcgccagcccccgctggccacg
FKRP-blk5-high-F	ccctacacgacgctcttccgatcttacacgatcctatgtggtgggcgtgctgg
FKRP-blk6-high-F	ccctacacgacgctcttccgatcttacacgatcaaccacttgcacgtggacct
FKRP-blk1-low-F	ccctacacgacgctcttccgatctaagtagagcacttggtaccggttctaga
FKRP-blk2-low-F	ccctacacgacgctcttccgatctaagtagaggcccgtggtggtggcagccg
FKRP-blk3-low-F	ccctacacgacgctcttccgatctaagtagaggccacggccaaccctgccag
FKRP-blk4-low-F	ccctacacgacgctcttccgatctaagtagaggccagcccccgctggccacg
FKRP-blk5-low-F	ccctacacgacgctcttccgatctaagtagagctatgtggtgggcgtgctgg
FKRP-blk6-low-F	ccctacacgacgctcttccgatctaagtagagaaccacttgcacgtggacct
FKRP-blk1-R	gactggagttcagacgtgtgctcttccgatctgggcgggtaggggagcgtgt
FKRP-blk2-R	gactggagttcagacgtgtgctcttccgatcttgacgttcagggccaggcac
FKRP-blk3-R	gactggagttcagacgtgtgctcttccgatctgccttccagcgcgcgtgggc
FKRP-blk4-R	gactggagttcagacgtgtgctcttccgatctgtagcgcacgcccgcagcct
FKRP-blk5-R	gactggagttcagacgtgtgctcttccgatcttgcgggggtagaagggccac
FKRP-blk6-R	gactggagttcagacgtgtgctcttccgatctcacttttcgggggatcctca
LARGE1-blk1-high-F	ccctacacgacgctcttccgatcttacacgatccacttggtaccggttctaga
LARGE1-blk2-high-F	ccctacacgacgctcttccgatcttacacgatccgcgaggtggaggaggagaa
LARGE1-blk3-high-F	ccctacacgacgctcttccgatcttacacgatccggatacaatgccagccggg
LARGE1-blk4-high-F	ccctacacgacgctcttccgatcttacacgatcgtctgatgaagcttgtcctg
LARGE1-blk5-high-F	ccctacacgacgctcttccgatcttacacgatcacaggggtgatcctgttact
LARGE1-blk6-high-F	ccctacacgacgctcttccgatcttacacgatccgtgtctgatctaaaggtca
LARGE1-blk7-high-F	ccctacacgacgctcttccgatcttacacgatcgagagcgcttcactgtccac
LARGE1-blk8-high-F	ccctacacgacgctcttccgatcttacacgatcatgagccgccacaacgtggg
LARGE1-blk9-high-F	ccctacacgacgctcttccgatcttacacgatcactgcgctaccggctgtcct
LARGE1-blk10-high-F	ccctacacgacgctcttccgatcttacacgatctaggctttggctggaacaaa
LARGE1-blk1-low-F	ccctacacgacgctcttccgatctaagtagagcacttggtaccggttctaga
LARGE1-blk2-low-F	ccctacacgacgctcttccgatctaagtagagcgcgaggtggaggaggagaa
LARGE1-blk3-low-F	ccctacacgacgctcttccgatctaagtagagcggatacaatgccagccggg
LARGE1-blk4-low-F	ccctacacgacgctcttccgatctaagtagaggtctgatgaagcttgtcctg

LARGE1-blk5-low-F	ccctacacgacgctcttccgatctaagtagagacaggggtgatcctgttact
LARGE1-blk6-low-F	ccctacacgacgctcttccgatctaagtagagcgtgtctgatctaaaggtca
LARGE1-blk7-low-F	ccctacacgacgctcttccgatctaagtagaggagagcgcttcactgtccac
LARGE1-blk8-low-F	ccctacacgacgctcttccgatctaagtagagatgagccgccacaacgtggg
LARGE1-blk9-low-F	ccctacacgacgctcttccgatctaagtagagactgcgctaccggctgtcct
LARGE1-blk10-low-F	ccctacacgacgctcttccgatctaagtagagtaggctttggctggaacaaa
LARGE1-blk1-R	gactggagttcagacgtgtgctcttccgatctgctgcctgcggagggcgcgg
LARGE1-blk2-R	gactggagttcagacgtgtgctcttccgatcttttgaccagggtgacgacat
LARGE1-blk3-R	gactggagttcagacgtgtgctcttccgatctttggcaggaagagtcttggt
LARGE1-blk4-R	gactggagttcagacgtgtgctcttccgatcttcttccgcagcttatccaga
LARGE1-blk5-R	gactggagttcagacgtgtgctcttccgatctcttgggggagttccagtgaa
LARGE1-blk6-R	gactggagttcagacgtgtgctcttccgatctaggaagtacaggtgggtgcg
LARGE1-blk7-R	gactggagttcagacgtgtgctcttccgatctccttgtacacgatgtggtag
LARGE1-blk8-R	gactggagttcagacgtgtgctcttccgatctctccgcttttgacttgggga
LARGE1-blk9-R	gactggagttcagacgtgtgctcttccgatctagctccatgatatgagccac
LARGE1-blk10-R	gactggagttcagacgtgtgctcttccgatctcacttttcgggggatccctа

Reaction conditions:

Q5 Reaction Buffer	10 μL	Step1	98 °C	Hot start
Q5 High GC Enhancer	10 μL	Step2	98 °C	3 mins
10 mM dNTPs	1 μL	Step3	98 °C	6 s
Q5 High-Fidelity DNA Polymerase	1 μL	Step4	Annealing temperature	15 s
10μM PCR2-F	2.5 μL	Step5	72 °C	7 s
10μM PCR2-R	2.5 μL	Step 3-5, 25 cycles		
gDNA	0.2-0.5 μg	Step6	72 °C	5 mins
Nuclease-Free Water	To 50 μL	Step7	12 °C	Infinite

Annealing temperature:

61 °C	LARGE1-blk1, LARGE1-blk4, LARGE1-blk6, LARGE1-blk7
64 °C	FKRP-blk1, LARGE1-blk5, LARGE1-blk9, LARGE1-blk10
66 °C	LARGE1-blk2, LARGE1-blk3, LARGE1-blk8
68 °C	FKRP-blk6
72 °C	FKRP-blk2, FKRP-blk3, FKRP-blk4, FKRP-blk5

PCR purification with NucleoSpin Gel and PCR Clean-Up Kit (Takara, 740609). Elute with 40 μL Nuclease-Free Water.

PCR3:

PCR3-F	aatgatacggcgaccaccgagatctacactctttccctacacgacgctcttccgatct
PCR3-R	caagcagaagacggcatacgagatcgcgcggtgtgactggagttcagacgtgtgctctt

Mix purified PCR2 products (200 ng each). Dilute the mixed sample to 11 ng/μL.

Q5 Reaction Buffer	10 μL	Step1	98 °C	Hot start
Q5 High GC Enhancer	10 μL	Step2	98 °C	3 mins
10 mM dNTPs	1 μL	Step3	98 °C	6 s
Q5 High-Fidelity DNA Polymerase	1 μL	Step4	72 °C	15 s
10μM PCR3-F	2.5 μL	Step5	72 °C	8 s
10μM PCR3-R	2.5 μL	Step 3-5, 25 cycles		
Mixed sample	23 μL	Step6	72 °C	5 mins
Set 3*50 μL reactions.		Step7	12 °C	Infinite

PCR purification with NucleoSpin Gel and PCR Clean-Up Kit (Takara, 740609). Elute with 50 μL Nuclease-Free Water for each column. The purified PCR3 product was used for the next generation sequencing. Amplicon-EZ service (GENEWIZ) was used to check the sample quality and coverage. The sample was then sequenced using the Hiseq X service (Psomagen; size selection also performed there).

Table 2.3.8 NGS library construction for SMuRF.

SMuRF score generation:

Enrichment of a variant (E_var) in a FACS group is calculated as a ratio of the count of the variant (c_var) to the total count (c_total) at the variant site:

$$E\_var = c\_var/c\_total$$

Enrichment of the WT (E_WT) is calculated separately for each block. E_WT is calculated as a ratio of the number of the reads without variant (r_WT) to the number of the reads with one or no variant (r_clean).

$$E\_WT = r\_WT/r\_clean$$

Relative enrichment (rE) is a ratio of the enrichment in the high-glycosylation group to the enrichment in the low-glycosylation group:

$$rE\_var = E\_var\_high/E\_var\_low$$

$$rE\_WT = E\_WT\_high/E\_WT\_low$$

The functional score of a variant is calculated as the ratio of its relative enrichment to that of the WT sequence in the corresponding block, and the SMuRF score is calculated as the log2 value of the functional score:

$$Functional\_score = rE\_var/rE\_WT$$

$$SMuRF = log2(Functional\_score)$$

Count of variants and reads were generated from raw sequencing data using the analytical pipeline deposited in the GitHub repository Gargamel. SMuRF scores were calculated using the scripts deposited in the GitHub repository Azrael.

Confidence score generation and classification:

In order to account for technical confounders, we have developed a confidence scoring system to assess the reliability of functional scores assigned to each variant. Our approach assumes that synonymous variants, which are not expected to have a functional effect, can serve as a null model. Hence, we expect the functional score for synonymous variants to be 1 (SMuRF=0). We have identified two key technical confounders: 1) the position of the variant in the block for the functional assay, and 2) the coverage (defined as the sum of "high" and "low" reads).

First, we developed a confidence score for each of these confounders. For the position in block, we binned the variants into groups, with each bin representing 10 base pairs. Within each bin, we took the mean of the functional score of all synonymous variants, and the confidence score per bin was then derived as follows:

$$Confidence\ (block\ position) = \frac{1}{mean(synoymous\ functional\ score)}$$

A confidence score that is closer to 1 indicates higher confidence/reliability. We employed a similar approach for the coverage-based confidence score; We binned the synonymous variants into groups representing every 5th percentile of the coverage distribution, and the per-bin confidence score was derived with the formula above.

Subsequently, we assigned both confidence scores to all variants in the testing set based on their position in the block and coverage. To integrate the effects of both confounding variables, the mean of both confidence scores for each variant was calculated. After this, a percentile-based confidence rank score was calculated based on the difference between the combined confidence score and 1 (which is taken to be the null, and further deviations from 1 indicate lower reliability). The final confidence rank score ranges from 0 to 1, with values closer to 1 indicating variants with higher confidence within the set. After which, the variants were assigned "LOW" confidence if their rank score is < 0.05, "MEDIUM" confidence if their rank score is ⩾ 0.05 and < 0.50, and "HIGH" confidence if their rank score is above 0.50.

Visualization of data on protein 3D structures:

Protein 3D structures from Protein Data Bank (PDB) were visualized using UCSF ChimeraX v1.3 [236]. The crystal structure of human FKRP (PDB:6KAM) [208] and the electron microscopy structure of LARGE1 (PDB:7UI7) [209] were used. Figures displaying domain locations or the log2 mean missense score per residue on 3D structures were generated using custom ChimeraX command files. Domain coordinates displayed are per Ortiz-Cordero *et al.* for FKRP [210], and Joseph *et al.* for LARGE1 [209]. The log2 of the mean missense score per residue was calculated using a custom Python script.

Immunofluorescence:

15 mm round Thermanox Coverslips (Thermo Scientific, 174969) were placed in the wells of 24-well plates. To coat the coverslips, 0.1% gelatin (Sigma-Aldrich, G9391) was added to the wells and immediately removed. After the coverslips were air-dried, 250k MB135 cells were resuspended in 0.5 mL growth medium and seeded into each well. One day after plating the cells, the medium was changed to the differentiation medium, and cells were differentiated for 3-7 days until myotubes were formed. The cells were washed with DPBS and fixed with 4% PFA (Sigma-Aldrich, 158127) for 10 mins at room temperature. The cells were blocked with 2% Bovine Serum Albumin (BSA, Sigma-Aldrich, A9647) at room temperature for 1 hr before undergoing incubation with the IIH6C4 antibody (1:200 in 2% BSA, Sigma-Aldrich, 05-593, discontinued) at 4 °C for 20 hrs. The cells were then washed with DPBS before undergoing incubation with the secondary antibody (1:100 in 2% BSA, Invitrogen, 31557) at room temperature for 2 hrs in the dark. Antifade Mounting Medium with DAPI (Vector Laboratories, H1500) was dropped onto Microscope Slides (Fisher Scientific, 22-037-246). The coverslips were washed again with DPBS and put onto the drops on the slides facedown and kept at room temperature for 30 mins in the dark. Pictures were taken with a Revolve ECHO microscope. (DO NOT use IIH6C4 antibody from Santa Cruz, sc-73586. An alternative IIH6C4 antibody may be acquired from Dr. Kevin Campbell.)

Packaging and infection of rVSV / ppVSV:

rVSV-LASV-GPC viral particles, ppVSVΔG-VSV-G viral particles, and the LASV-GPC plasmid were obtained from Dr. Melinda Brindley's group. To package ppVSV-

LASV-GPC viral particles, HEK293T cells were transfected with the LASV-GPC plasmid and then transduced with ppVSVΔG-VSV-G viral particles. The resulting particles were referred to as ppVSV-LASV-GPC-Generation1. A new batch of LASV-GPC transfected HEK293T cells were subsequently transduced with ppVSV-LASV-GPC-Generation1 to produce ppVSV-LASV-GPC-Generation2, reducing residual VSV-G in the pseudotyped particles. Similarly, later generations can be packaged. The experiments in this study utilized ppVSV-LASV-GPC-Generation2 and 3. The 50% tissue culture infectious dose (TCID50) of the VSV was determined using the Spearman-Karber method [237,238]. Detailed ppVSV packaging protocol can be found in Table 2.3.9. Lentiviral transduction and blasticidin drug selection were performed in the same manner as those in the FACS assay. Afterwards, cells were divided into two groups (~1M cells each): a no-infection group and an infection group. rVSV infection was conducted at an approximate MOI of 0.5. NH_4Cl (Sigma-Aldrich, A9434, final conc. 5mM) was added during the infection and subsequent recovery. After 60 hours of infection, the medium was replaced, and the cells were allowed to recover for 12 hours before harvesting. ppVSV infection was performed at an approximate MOI of 1~3, and the infected cells were recovered to ~1M prior to harvesting.

General information:
The LASV-GPC plasmid and the ppVSVΔG-VSV-G viral particles were obtained from Dr. Melinda Brindley's group.
The ppVSVΔG-VSV-G viral particles carry a GFP-coding sequence in their genomes, which can be used to determine the TCID50 (tissue culture infectious dose which will infect 50% of the cell monolayers).
TCID50 of the viral particles were experimentally determined using a protocol provided by Dr. Melinda Brindley. The protocol was based on the Spearman-Karber method [237,238].
To calculate multiplicity of infection (MOI) based on TCID50, a working estimate was adopted: $plaque\ forming\ units\ (pfu) = 0.5 * TCID50$

$MOI = pfu\ of\ virus\ /\ number\ of\ cells$	
Exercise standard caution when handling viral particles!	
Biosafety Level 2 (BSL-2) for activities with materials and cultures known or reasonably expected to contain VSV.	
Making ppVSV-LASV-GPC-Generation1:	
Day 0	Seed HEK293T cells in a well of a 6-well plate.
Day 1	Perform Lipofectamine 3000 (Invitrogen, L3000001) transfection per manufacturer's instruction.
	HEK293T should reach 70%-90% confluency.
	4 μg LASV-GPC plasmid was used to transfect the cells.
Day 2	24 hrs after transfection, ppVSVΔG-VSV-G (MOI=0.5) was added to the well.
	The cell number is estimated to be ~2 M. Use this number to decide the viral dose.
	1 hr after adding the ppVSVΔG-VSV-G, the medium was removed, the well was washed with DPBS (Gibco, 14190144), and fresh medium was added to the well.
Day 3	Collect the newly generated viral particles, *i.e.*, ppVSV-LASV-GPC-Generation1, and titrate its titer.
Making ppVSV-LASV-GPC-Generation2:	
Day 0	Seed 6M HEK293T cells in a 10-cm dish.
Day 1	Perform Lipofectamine 3000 (Invitrogen, L3000001) transfection per manufacturer's instruction.
	30 μg LASV-GPC plasmid was used to transfect the cells.
Day 2	24 hrs after transfection, ppVSV-LASV-GPC-Generation1 (MOI=0.1) was added to the well.
	The cell number is estimated to be ~12 M. Use this number to decide the viral dose.
	1 hr after adding the ppVSV-LASV-GPC-Generation1, the medium was removed, the well was washed with DPBS (Gibco, 14190144), and fresh medium was added to the well.
Day 3	Collect the newly generated viral particles, *i.e.*, ppVSV-LASV-GPC-Generation2, and titrate its titer.
Using ppVSV-LASV-GPC-Generation2, ppVSV-LASV-GPC-Generation3 can be packaged similarly as ppVSV-LASV-GPC-Generation2.	
NGS library construction for VSV-related experiments was performed using a procedure similar to that outlined in Table 2.3.8. The "high" primers were utilized for the infected groups, while the primers provided below were used for the non-infected groups.	
FKRP-blk1-noinf-F	ccctacacgacgctcttccgatctcctacgtcacttggtaccggttctaga
FKRP-blk2-noinf-F	ccctacacgacgctcttccgatctcctacgtgcccgtggtggtggcagccg
FKRP-blk3-noinf-F	ccctacacgacgctcttccgatctcctacgtgccacggccaaccctgccag
FKRP-blk4-noinf-F	ccctacacgacgctcttccgatctcctacgtgccagccccgctggccacg
FKRP-blk5-noinf-F	ccctacacgacgctcttccgatctcctacgtctatgtggtgggcgtgctgg
FKRP-blk6-noinf-F	ccctacacgacgctcttccgatctcctacgtaaccacttgcacgtggacct
LARGE1-blk1-noinf-F	ccctacacgacgctcttccgatctcctacgtcacttggtaccggttctaga
LARGE1-blk2-noinf-F	ccctacacgacgctcttccgatctcctacgtcgcgaggtggaggaggagaa
LARGE1-blk3-noinf-F	ccctacacgacgctcttccgatctcctacgtcggatacaatgccagccggg
LARGE1-blk4-noinf-F	ccctacacgacgctcttccgatctcctacgtgtctgatgaagcttgtcctg
LARGE1-blk5-noinf-F	ccctacacgacgctcttccgatctcctacgtacaggggtgatcctgttact
LARGE1-blk6-noinf-F	ccctacacgacgctcttccgatctcctacgtcgtgtctgatctaaaggtca
LARGE1-blk7-noinf-F	ccctacacgacgctcttccgatctcctacgtgagagcgcttcactgtccac
LARGE1-blk8-noinf-F	ccctacacgacgctcttccgatctcctacgtatgagccgccacaacgtggg
LARGE1-blk9-noinf-F	ccctacacgacgctcttccgatctcctacgtactgcgctaccggctgtcct
LARGE1-blk10-noinf-F	ccctacacgacgctcttccgatctcctacgttaggctttggctggaacaaa

Table 2.3.9 ppVSV packaging protocol and NGS library construction for VSV-related experiments.

Protein extraction and quantitation:

Ice-cold protein extraction lysis buffer made by adding 10 μL of protease inhibitor cocktail (Sigma Aldrich, P8340-1ML) to every 1 mL of RIPA lysis and extraction buffer (Pierce, PI89900) was used to treat the cells. After 15 minutes of rocking incubation on ice, the samples were centrifuged for 30 minutes at 16,000 × g at 4 °C in a refrigerated centrifuge (Eppendorf, 5404). The supernatant was transferred to a clean 1.5 mL microcentrifuge tube for following steps.

Protein was quantitated using the BioRad DC Assay II kit (BioRad, 5000112). Using the BSA reagent from the kit, seven standards are prepared from 0-1.5 mg/mL in the protein extraction lysis buffer from above for creating a standard curve. Measurements were done according to the instruction manual, and absorbances at 750nm were read on a plate reader (BioRad, #1681135). Concentration is calculated relative to the standard curve.

SDS-PAGE and western blotting:

Appropriate amount of protein extraction lysis buffer from above was added into each protein sample (~10 μg) to balance the samples to achieve an equal volume. 4x Laemlli (BioRad, 1610747) was supplemented with 10% b-mercaptoethanol. 1 μL of this supplemented buffer was then added to every 3 μL of the balanced sample. Samples were mixed by a brief vortex and then heated at ~95°C on a heat block (BioRad, 1660571) for 5 minutes. Samples were cooled down on ice and then centrifuged briefly at max speed to ensure equal loading (Eppendorf, 5404).

3.5 μL of PageRuler Plus prestained protein ladder (ThermoFisher Scientific, 26619) and all of the samples were then loaded onto a 4-15% mini-protean TGX stain free protein gel (*e.g.*, BioRad, 4568084) that had been placed into a Mini-PROTEAN tetra cell electrophoresis system (BioRad, 1658000). SDS-PAGE was performed at 120V for ~60 minutes using a PowerPac HC power supply (BioRad, 1645052). Upon completion of the SDS-PAGE, the gel was removed and transferred onto a nitrocellulose membrane (BioRad, 1704158) by the TransBlot Turbo System (BioRad, 1704150EDU) using the 7-minute transfer program (2.5 A constant, up to 25 V variable).

Vinculin was used as a loading control. Hence, the membrane was cut at the correct position for separate FKRP and vinculin WBs. Membrane blocking buffer was made of 5% Omniblock non-fat dry milk (American Bio, AB10109-00100) in 1× TBS-Tween 20 (TBS-T). The membrane pieces were then blocked for 1 hour in membrane blocking buffer separately.

Primary Anti-FKRP antibody (Abcam, ab220059) was made up 1:1,000 in membrane blocking buffer. Primary Anti-Vinculin antibody (Sigma Aldrich, V9131-100 μl) was made up 1:80,000 in membrane blocking buffer. The membrane pieces were incubated in the corresponding primary antibodies overnight at 4°C whilst rocking to equally distribute antibody (BenchRocker 2D Genesee Scientific, 31-201).

The following day, the membrane pieces were washed 5 times for 5 minutes in TBS-T and incubated in corresponding secondary antibodies for 2 hours at room temperature. Anti-rabbit HRP conjugated secondary antibody (Cell Signaling Technology, 7074S) was used for FKRP at 1:2,000 in membrane blocking buffer. Anti-mouse HRP conjugated secondary antibody (Cell Signaling Technology, 7076S) was used for vinculin at 1:2,000 in membrane blocking buffer.

Membrane pieces were washed again 5 times for 5 mins at room temperature in TBS-T prior to developing with Clarity Max ECL substrate (BioRad, 1705062) or Clarity ECL substrate (BioRad, 1705060). Using the Chemidoc Imaging system (BioRad, 12005606), both chemiluminescent and colorimetric images were taken to observe protein expression and size of bands.

Statistics:

Two-sided Wilcoxon tests were performed with the "ggsignif" R package. Spearman's rank correlation coefficients were calculated with the "cor.test" function in R.

Data availability:

FFC and FACS datasets were made available on FlowRepository (FR-FCM-Z6LL, FR-FCM-Z6LM, FR-FCM-Z6LN, FR-FCM-Z6LP, FR-FCM-Z6LQ, FR-FCM-Z6LR, FR-FCM-Z6LX). NGS raw data were deposited to Sequence Read Archive (SRA) of the National Center for Biotechnology Information (NCBI) (accession: PRJNA993285). All scripts used in this project can be found on GitHub (https://github.com/leklab). Scripts in the Balthazar repository were used for oligo design and other pre-SMuRF experiments. Analytical pipeline in the Gargamel repository was used for processing the raw NGS data. Scripts in the Azrael repository were used for generating SMuRF scores and downstream analyses.

2.4 Future Expansion of SMuRF

When we initially embarked on the establishment of SMuRF, our vision encompassed the creation of a versatile workflow capable of integrating various saturation mutagenesis techniques and diverse functional assays for different genes, analogous to assembling Lego bricks. This section serves as a preview, highlighting the potential inclusion of additional saturation mutagenesis methods and functional assays within the SMuRF workflow, along with our primary accomplishments in implementing these methods.

2.4.1 Prime editing screen

Although the PALS-C cloning- and lentiviral delivery-based saturation mutagenesis method proved to be cost-effective and straightforward for our projects involving *FKRP* and *LARGE1*, one of its drawbacks cannot be easily overlooked. This disadvantage stems from the fact that exogenous viral gene expression removes the entire endogenous genomic context, including regulatory elements such as enhancers and promoters, as well as introns and splicing-related elements. Integrating an endogenous saturation mutagenesis method into the SMuRF workflow could broaden its coverage of a wider range of molecular biological events underlying disease mechanisms.

Currently, the predominant endogenous saturation mutagenesis method in the field is saturation genome editing (SGE), which relies on CRISPR-mediated cutting and homology-directed repair (HDR) [24,239-242]. Variants are introduced into the HDR templates to achieve saturation mutagenesis.

Recently, a novel endogenous saturation mutagenesis method based on Prime Editing (PE) has emerged [229] and holds the potential to be a more favorable alternative to SGE. This judgement is founded on the subsequent considerations: Firstly, in SGE, saturation mutagenesis relies on generating double-stranded breaks (DSBs), which raises concerns about off-target effects. Secondly, when aiming to perform SGE over a large region, the most cost-effective approach involves dividing the task into multiple jobs, each with a corresponding gRNA targeting a smaller region [239]. However, this could increase the labor requirement.

On the other hand, PE-based saturation mutagenesis addresses these issues in two aspects. One, PE utilizes the Cas9 nickase rather than a nuclease, which reduces the off-target indels associated with DSBs [243,244]. Two, since the genome-targeting sequence and the reverse transcriptase template are combined in the same gRNA sequence in PE, even when targeting multiple loci, the experiments can be performed in a pooled manner.

With the advantages of PE in mind, we began establishing a workflow for PE saturation mutagenesis for *FKTN*, another gene involved in α-DG glycosylation, in collaboration with our collaborators at SickKids. Both SGE and PE screens are known for their relatively low efficiency, relatively high cost, and dependence on genomic context [245-247]. In the process of developing the *FKTN* PE screen, we are also working to optimize the experimental procedures to address these issues, aiming to make the PE screen method more accessible for more labs in the rare disease field.

The initial step involved establishing a platform cell line, specifically a *MLH1*-knockout (KO), *FKTN*-haploidized, and inducible PE-incorporated monoclonal MB135 cell line (Fig. 2.4.1.1a). *MLH1*, a gene associated with DNA mismatch repair [248,249], was firstly knocked out using CRISPR ribonucleoprotein (RNP) in MB135 (Fig. 2.4.1.1b and Table 2.4.1.2), based on prior research suggesting that its disruption could enhance PE editing efficiency [250,251]. Subsequently, *FKTN* haploidization was performed using CRISPR RNP to delete one allele of the gene (Fig. 2.4.1.1c,d and Table 2.4.1.3), which is another well-established strategy to enhance PE editing efficiency [229]. Next, we utilized the Sleeping Beauty transposon system [252] to integrate the doxycycline-inducible PE construct (a gift from Dr. Zhenya Ivakine) into the genome (Fig. 2.4.1.1e and Table 2.4.1.4). Currently, we are actively evaluating the monoclonal cell lines (Fig. 2.4.1.1e), and selecting the most optimal candidate.

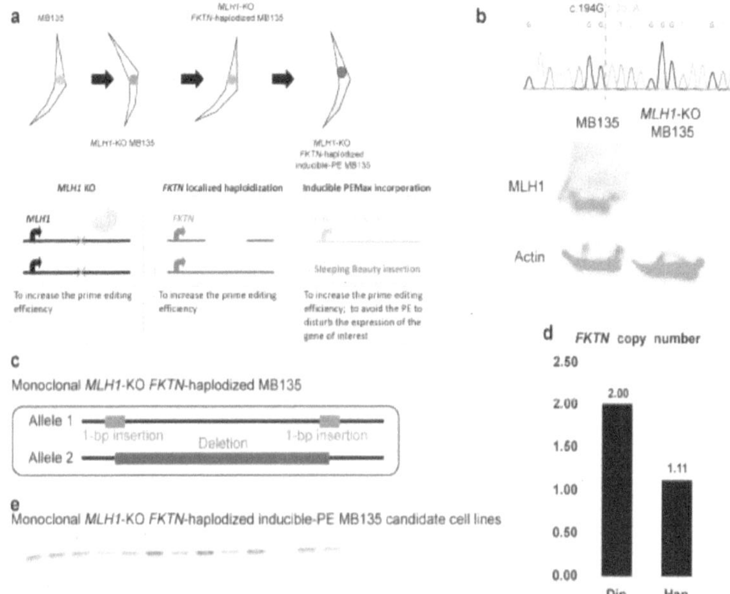

Fig. 2.4.1.1 Development of a platform cell line for *FKTN* PE Saturation Mutagenesis. a, Generating the platform cell line. Each arrow represents an engineering step, with a monoclonal line established at each step for subsequent steps. PEMax: an optimized prime editor [251]. **b,** Sanger sequencing and WB validations for the monoclonal *MLH1*-KO MB135 cell line. **c,** 3-reaction genotyping (Table 2.4.1.3) confirmed that this monoclonal line was indeed haploidized at the *FKTN* locus. Sanger sequencing identified two insertions on the allele that was not deleted. **d,** TaqMan real-time PCR confirmed the successful haploidization of *FKTN* without the insertion of its sequence into other loci of the genome. Dip.: *MLH1*-KO MB135. Hap.: *MLH1*-KO *FKTN*-haploidized MB135. The *FKTN* copy number was set to 2 for Dip.. *FKRP* primers and probe were used as a control. **e,** Genotyping confirmed the successful incorporation of PE in the monoclonal *MLH1*-KO *FKTN*-haploidized inducible PE-incorporated MB135 cell lines.

gRNA for *MLH1*-KO	aagacaatggcaccgggatc
Genotyping primer F for *MLH1*-KO	tgtatgagcctgtaagacaaaggaa
Genotyping primer R for *MLH1*-KO	catccatattgaagccttcctgaac
MLH1-KO mutation	Homozygous c.195-201 del
MLH1 antibody	Abcam, ab92312
Actin antibody	Proteintech, 66009-1-lg
***FKTN* haploidization-related GRCh38 coordinates:**	
FKTN deleted allele deletion	1 A substituting chr9 105557700(A)-105656064(A)
FKTN remaining allele insertion 1	1 T between chr9:105557700 (A) and 105557701 (G)
FKTN remaining allele insertion 2	1 G between chr9: 105656066 (G) and 105656067 (C)

Table 2.4.1.2 Materials for *MLH1* knockout and subsequent validation.

gRNA1 for *FKTN* haploidization	GATACAATTAGTAGAGCTAG
gRNA2 for *FKTN* haploidization	CCCAAGTATCACACGAGGCG

Genotyping primer F1	TTAAACTGGAGGGCAACAGG
Genotyping primer R1	ACTCTTGTCGCATCCTCACC
Genotyping primer F2	TGCAGATTTCAGACCACACC
Genotyping primer R2	GTATGGCTCAGCGAGAGACC
How to use the genotyping primers:	
F1 & R2	PCR band on gel indicates at least one allele of *FKTN* was deleted
F1 & R1	PCR band on gel indicates at least one allele of *FKTN* was NOT deleted
F2 & R2	
DNA was extracted from the cells and used for Taqman real-time PCR:	
Probes and PrimeTime Gene Expression Master Mix were ordered from IDT	
FKTN real-time PCR-F	CCTAAGGGAGTTTGCTGTGG
FKTN real-time PCR-R	AGATACTGGGCCAACACAGG
FKTN probe	/5SUN/CA CAG TGA A/ZEN/T TAT GAA TAT CTG TCT TGT CCT CT/3IABkFQ/
FKRP real-time PCR-F	TGGGCATCTACTTGGAGGAC
FKRP real-time PCR-R	TTGCTTTCGCTGTACTGCAC
FKRP probe	/56-FAM/AC CGC CTT C/ZEN/T CCC ATA CGA AGC /3IABkFQ/

Table 2.4.1.3 Materials for *FKTN* haploidization and subsequent validation.

PE genotyping F	tccacctgtttaccctgacc
PE genotyping R	gttccttgcttgtttcatgc
PE qPCR F	acctgggatatagggcatcc
PE qPCR R	atgaacagcctgcaaaatcc

Table 2.4.1.4 Primers for validation of PE incorporation.

At the same time, we are currently developing a cloning method to create a lentiviral plasmid library of PE gRNAs (pegRNAs), which will enable us to achieve saturation mutagenesis for *FKTN* (Fig. 2.4.1.5). Importantly, the PE technique allows us to perform saturation mutagenesis not only for single nucleotides and single amino acids but also for small insertions, deletions, duplications, and inversions. The plan is to integrate the soon-to-be established PE saturation mutagenesis method for *FKTN* with the ppVSV assay that has been developed in the *FKRP* project. Our initial step will involve optimizing the experimental setups for this combination using several *FKTN* variants with ClinVar reports (Table 2.4.1.6). Subsequently, we aim to develop this into a DMS workflow for *FKTN*. Our goal is to enhance our understanding of the functional landscape of *FKTN*, as well as contributing a novel methodology to the ongoing quest for a comprehensive Variant Effects Atlas.

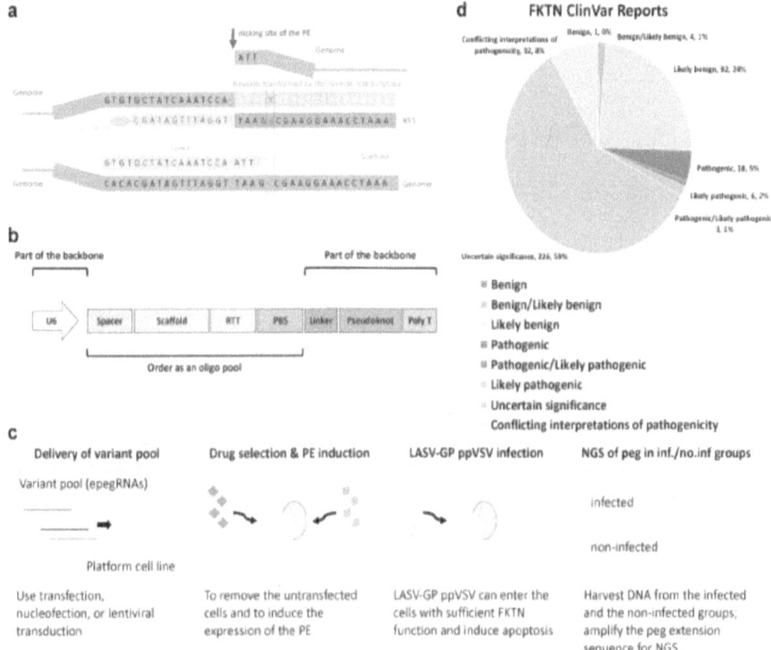

Fig. 2.4.1.5 Establishing the PE saturation mutagenesis-based DMS workflow for *FKTN*. a, An example of the PE saturation mutagenesis at a given site. d: t or a or g. h: a or t or c. **b,** A schematic diagram of the epeg construct. epeg: engineered pegRNA [253]. **c,** The proposed DMS workflow for *FKTN*. **d,** *FKTN* variants are poorly interpreted (Coding single nucleotide variants; ClinVar results July 19th, 2022).

Variants	ClinVar	Spacer	peg extension	PAM	GMAF
c.139C>T (p.Arg47Ter)	Pathogenic	GTGTGCTATC AAATCCAATT	AAATCCAAAGGAAGC tGAATTGGATTTGAT AGC	disrupted	NA
c.346C>T (p.Gln116Ter)	Pathogenic	CACTTACCTC ATTCTTCCAT	GCACTGtAGTATCAC CTATGGAAGAATGAG GTA	intact	NA
c.895A>C (p.Ser299Arg)	Uncertain significance	ACAAATTGGG AGTACCATTC	GTTCCACgGCTCAGC CAGAATGGTACTCCC AAT	intact	NA
c.1325A>G (p.Asn442Ser)	Conflicting interpretations	ATTCCATTGG GTTGCACATT	GGAAGCGCTCTCCT CCCAgTGTGCAACCC AATG	intact	NA
c.373G>A (p.Gly125Ser)	Benign/Likely benign	TTTGATGCTT CTTTGGTTCT	TCCGAAACCAGCaTT CCTAGAACCAAAGAA	disrupted	0.03714

			GCAT		
c.1026C>A (p.Leu342=)	Benign/Likely benign	TTCCCAAATT TGTGTTTGAG	AGGATGCAGGACTT CCGCTaAAACACAAA TTTG	intact	0.17832

Table 2.4.1.6 ClinVar *FKTN* variants for proof-of-concept cloning. GMAF: Global minor allele frequency. When designing pegRNAs for the saturation mutagenesis library, the following pegRNA sequences should be removed: (1) the ones with a C as the first base of the peg extension and (2) the ones with a homopolymer T stretch. The pegRNA sequences were designed with PrimeDesign [254].

2.4.2 Mitochondrial genome editing

Mitochondria are the primary producers of cellular energy and hold a pivotal role in various cellular functions such as signaling pathways, redox homeostasis, immune response, and metabolic regulation [255-257]. Disruptions in mtDNA can lead to both mitochondrial and cellular dysfunctions, contributing to diverse human disorders [258-261]. However, despite its critical significance in health and disease, the consequences of mtDNA variants remain largely unknown. To date, DMS studies for mtDNA have been notably absent. However, we believe that recent advancements in biotechnological tools have equipped us with the necessary resources to conduct such studies, and this potential development could serve as a valuable addition to the comprehensive Variant Effects Atlas.

In fact, a functional assay known as the "glucose-galactose" assay has long been established for mitochondria [262263], and it can be easily adapted for the evaluation of mtDNA variants [264]. Fast growing cells mainly rely on glycolysis thus are unaffected by mitochondrial impairment in glucose medium. Galactose medium forces the cells to shift the energy metabolism from glycolysis to oxidative phosphorylation, making them more sensitive to mitochondrial impairment (Fig. 2.4.2.1b). Therefore, by quantifying the enrichment of an mtDNA variant before and after changing the medium from glucose to galactose, we can assess the functional effects of this variant. There seems to be no hindrance to utilizing this assay in a pooled manner. However, several rounds of optimization will undoubtedly be necessary to achieve optimal sensitivity.

With that aspect being established, the remaining puzzle to solve is achieving saturation mutagenesis for mtDNA. Notably, the recent development of transcription activator-like effector (TALE)-based mtDNA base editors has significantly enhanced the efficiency and applicability of mitochondrial genome editing [265-267]. Indeed, in our experiment, we attained remarkably high levels of base editing in the mitochondrial genome through the utilization of the DdCBE base editor. This system incorporates TALE proteins and a double-stranded DNA-specific cytidine deaminase (DddA) to introduce C•G-to-T•A editing [265] (Fig. 2.4.2.1a).

DddA was originally an inter-bacterial toxin with inherent toxicity to human cells. To mitigate this toxicity, the toxin was split into two inactive halves during the development of DdCBE [268]. The restoration of deamination activity would occur solely upon their adjacent assembly on target DNA, resembling the reconstitution of dsDNA nuclease activity in TALEN through the assembly of FokI monomers [269]. This strategy, though ingenious at the time, presents significant challenges when attempting to adapt it for saturation mutagenesis due to the requirement of two TALEs, which considerably complicates the cloning processes. Fortunately, a recent study has successfully developed non-toxic, full-length DddA variants that can be utilized to create monomeric DdCBEs (mDdCBEs) [270].

With this recent advancement, the prospect of achieving saturation mutagenesis in the mitochondrial genome is becoming clearer. However, several challenges still need to be addressed before this can be realized. One such challenge is finding a way to perform mitochondrial saturation mutagenesis in a pooled manner without compromising the sensitivity of the functional assay. This is particularly complex due to the presence of multiple mitochondria within each cell. More preliminary experiments are required to establish such a workflow. However, once established, the DMS in mitochondria will undoubtedly lead to a significant improvement in our understanding of mtDNA variants.

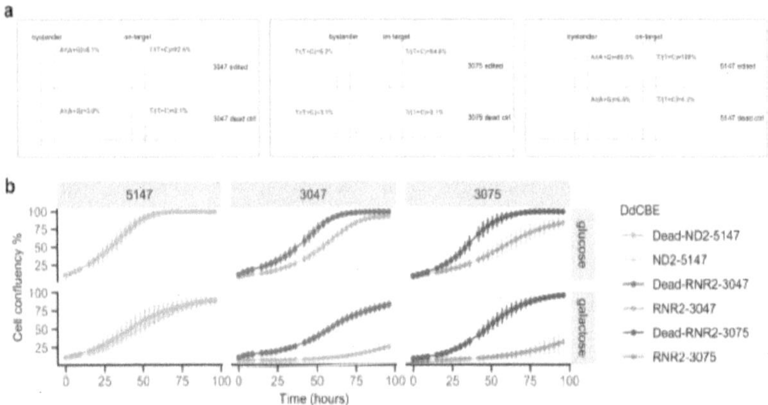

Fig. 2.4.2.1 Establishing a DMS workflow for mtDNA variants. a, HEK293T cells transfected with base editor DdCBE to introduce a synonymous m.5147G>A in MT-ND2, or m.3047G>A and m.3075G>A in a highly constrained region in MT-RNR2. The dead DdCBE controls are also shown. For the transfection,150 k cells were plated in a well of a 12-well plate one day prior to the Lipofectamine 3000 transfection (Invitrogen, L3000001). 2 μg left plasmid (or dead left plasmid) and 2 μg right plasmid were transfected per condition (Table 2.4.2.2) per manufacturer's manual. FACS (GFP & mCherry channel) and/or drug selection [~5μg/mL blasticidin (Gibco, A1113903) and ~1μg/mL puromycin (Gibco, A1113803)] was performed to enrich the dual-plasmid-transfected cells. Drug selection after live cell sorting achieved the highest pooled editing efficiency. Additionally, transfection conducted without the presence of Anti-anti in the medium significantly enhances the efficiency. Chromatograms: red, T; blue, C; green, A; black, G. The figures depict the Sanger sequencing results of the targeted PCR products (Table 2.4.2.3). Editing efficiencies were quantified using the EditR tools based on the Sanger sequencing results [271]. Additionally, PacBio long-read sequencing of the long-read PCR products was performed and validated the editing efficiencies. **b,** Growth curves in transfected HEK293T cells cultured in glucose or galactose (which requires mitochondrial energy generation). Measurements were done using an Incucyte S3 live-cell imaging system. Values and error bars reflect the mean ± s.e.m. of n = 4 (ND2-5147, RNR2-3047) or n = 5 (RNR2-3075) independent biological replicates. [Base editing efficiencies across replicates were 66-96%

for ND2-5147, 93-98% for RNR2-3047, and 93-96% for RNR2-3075]. The galactose medium was made by mixing DMEM (no glucose; Gibco, 11966025), galactose (4.5 g/L) 10% FBS and 1 × Anti-anti. For the glucose-galactose growth assay, approximately 12k to 16k cells were seeded per well in a 48-well plate (Falcon, 353078) to achieve an even distribution and ~10-15% seeding confluency. 3 wells were plated per treatment per medium condition. After allowing the cells to attach to the plate in glucose medium (~1-3 hours), the medium was replaced with the corresponding fresh medium for both glucose and galactose groups. The Incucyte S3 (Sartorius) captured 9-16 images per well every 3 hours over a span of 96 hours. Subsequently, the confluency in each image was quantified using the software installed in the Incucyte machine.

Name	Purpose	Resistance	Fluorescence	Backbone
p3047-L	3047 G->A	BSD	mCherry	Addgene, 179682
p3047-R	3047 G->A	PuroR	eGFP	Engineered from Addgene, 179686
p3047-dead-L	No-editing ctrl	BSD	mCherry	Addgene, 179683
p3075-L	3075 G->A	BSD	mCherry	Addgene, 179682
p3075-R	3075 G->A	PuroR	eGFP	Engineered from Addgene, 179686
p3075-dead-L	No-editing ctrl	BSD	mCherry	Addgene, 179683
p5147-L	5147 G->A	BSD	mCherry	Addgene, 179682
p5147-R	5147 G->A	PuroR	eGFP	Engineered from Addgene, 179686
p5147-dead-L	No-editing ctrl	BSD	mCherry	Addgene, 179683

Table 2.4.2.2 Plasmids generated in the initial stage of establishing a DMS workflow for mtDNA variants. The codon-optimized transcription activator-like effector (TALE) constructs were synthesized using either the gBlocks service from IDT or the GeneArt service from Invitrogen. Addgene plasmids 179682, 179683, and 179686 were gifts from David Liu.

3047-3075-F	TCACCAGTCAAAGCGAACTACT			
3047-3075-R	GGGTACAATGAGGAGTAGGAGGTT			
5147-F	CCAAATCTCTCCCTCACTAAACG	Difficult template for Sanger sequencing		
5147-R	AGGTAGGAGTAGCGTGGTAAG	Difficult template for Sanger sequencing		
Targeted PCR was performed with the following conditions:				
Q5 Rxn buffer	10 μL	1	98 °C	hot start
Q5 Enh buffer	10 μL	2	98 °C	3 mins
Q5 polymerase (NEB, M0491S)	1 μL	3	98 °C	8 s
		4	Annealing temperature*	15 s
10 mM dNTPs	1 μL	5	72 °C	15 s
DNA extracted from cells	400 ng	6	Repeat 3-5 for 34 more cycles	
10 μM F primer	2.5 μL	7	72 °C	5 mins
10 μM R primer	2.5 μL	8	12 °C	Forever
Water	To 50 μL	*3047-3075: 67 °C; 5147: 66 °C		
Long-read PCR F1	CAGATATCAATAAGACATCACGATGGATCACA			
Long-read PCR F2	GTGCACGTAATAAGACATCACGATGGATCACA			
Long-read PCR F3	AGAACATTAATAAGACATCACGATGGATCACA			
Long-read PCR F4	AGTTATAAAATAAGACATCACGATGGATCACA			
Long-read PCR F5	GTCTTCTTAATAAGACATCACGATGGATCACA			
Long-read PCR F6	TTAAACACAATAAGACATCACGATGGATCACA			
Long-read PCR F7	AATCTTCCAATAAGACATCACGATGGATCACA			
Long-read PCR F8	TGCTCAGTAATAAGACATCACGATGGATCACA			
Long-read PCR R1	AGGGTTGCTAAGGGGAACGTGTGGGCTATTT			
Long-read PCR R2	CATGTGGATAAGGGGAACGTGTGGGCTATTT			

Long-read PCR R3	GATTCCACTAAGGGGAACGTGTGGGCTATTT			
Long-read PCR R4	TACGATTCTAAGGGGAACGTGTGGGCTATTT			
Long-read PCR R5	GGTACATGTAAGGGGAACGTGTGGGCTATTT			
Long-read PCR R6	GTTATCGTTAAGGGGAACGTGTGGGCTATTT			
Long-read PCR R7	TATTGCTATAAGGGGAACGTGTGGGCTATTT			
Long-read PCR R8	GCCAGCCTTAAGGGGAACGTGTGGGCTATTT			
Long-read PCR was performed with the following conditions:				
DNA extracted from cells	400 ng	1	98 °C	hot start
Phusion Master Mix with GC Buffer (2X) (Thermo Scientific, F532S)	25 μL	2	98 °C	30 s
		3	98 °C	30 s
10 μM F primer	2.5 μL	4	63 °C	30 s
10 μM R primer	2.5 μL	5	72 °C	9 mins
DMSO	1.5 μL	6	Repeat 3-5 for 9 more cycles	
Water	To 50 μL	7	98 °C	30 s
Purification, size selection, and long-read sequencing were performed at Yale Center for Genome Analysis (YCGA).		8	67 °C	30 s
		9	72 °C	9 mins
		10	Repeat 7-9 for 9 more cycles	
		11	72 °C	10 mins
		12	4 °C	Forever

Table 2.4.2.3 Primers used in the initial stage of establishing a DMS workflow for mtDNA variants. Red: barcodes.

Chapter 3: Accelerating the development of gene therapy in precision medicine

3.1 Introduction to Duchenne Muscular Dystrophy (DMD) and the exon-1 deletion

Duchenne muscular dystrophy (DMD) and Becker muscular dystrophy (BMD) are both X-linked genetic disorders characterized by muscle weakness and wasting. They are caused by mutations in the dystrophin gene *DMD*, a large structural gene consisting of 2.4 Mb genomic DNA with 79 exons [272,273].

In DMD, the mutations primarily consist of nonsense or frameshift mutations, leading to a complete absence or significantly reduced levels of functional dystrophin protein [274]. Notably, the missense variant L54R is also associated with DMD, potentially due to its impact on focal adhesion tension and mechanotransduction [275]. DMD, as a severe form of muscular dystrophy, often leads to loss of ambulation and significant health complications [276]. In contrast, BMD is a milder form characterized by mutations such as missense mutations [277], nonsense mutations that lead to exon skipping [278], or in-frame deletions/duplications [279]. These mutations generally lead to a shortened or partially functional dystrophin protein. BMD typically has a later onset, slower disease progression, and a more favorable prognosis compared to DMD [280]. Both DMD and BMD share a common cellular pathophysiology, where the absence or dysfunction of dystrophin compromises the integrity of the dystrophin-glycoprotein complex (DGC) [272]. DGC is essential for maintaining the structural integrity of muscle cells and preventing damage to the sarcolemma during muscle contraction [281].

A patient, referred to as Patient1 hereafter, was diagnosed with DMD in the first decade of life, with loss of independent ambulation occurring in his second decade of life. He had progressive decline in his upper extremity function with increasing cardiopulmonary dysfunction. A skeletal muscle biopsy revealed patchy dystrophin immunostaining, which was shown to be approximately 3% of control muscle by western blot (Fig. 3.1.1a-c). Whole genome sequencing revealed a hemizygous deletion of approximately 30.7 kb (GRCh38 chrX: 33,194,894-33,225,637), resulting in the loss of exon 1 of the muscle isoform (Fig. 3.1.1d).

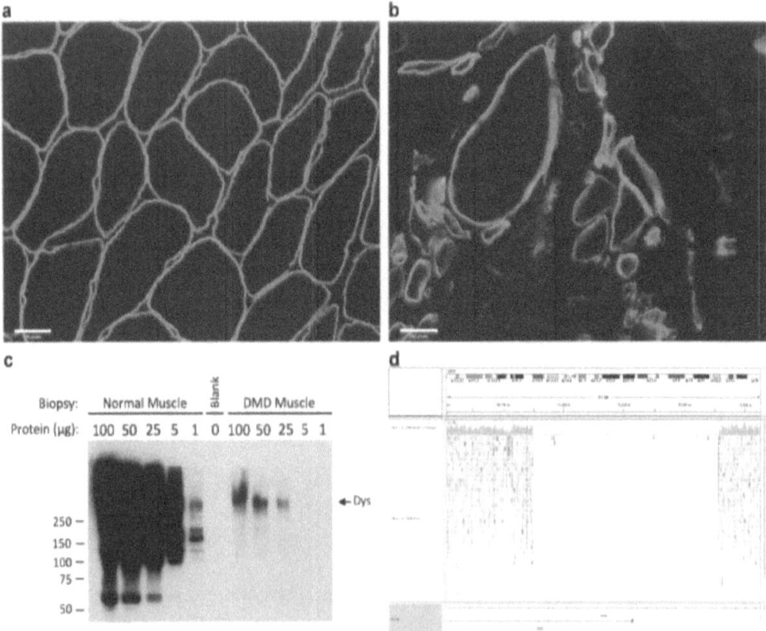

Fig. 3.1.1 **Diagnosis of Patient1 with *Dp427m* exon1 deletion.** Frozen muscle tissue section from a de-identified unaffected individual (**a**) and Patient1 (**b**) immunostained for dystrophin. Dystrophin staining is visible at the myofiber sarcolemma in the unaffected control sample and also in several myofibers of different sizes in the proband. The positive staining was detected using antibodies to the dystrophin rod domain and C-terminus (CAP 6-10 antibody generated in Kunkel Lab). **c**, Western blot of normal and DMD patient quadricep muscle biopsies shows significantly diminished dystrophin expression in DMD patient compared to normal muscle. WB quantification indicates ~2.9% dystrophin protein expression in

DMD patient compared to normal muscle. WB signals were quantified by pixel density using ImageJ. **d**, Whole genome sequencing reveals a ~30.7 kb hemizygous deletion (GRCh38 chrX: 33,194,894-33,225,637) encompassing the promoter and exon 1 of the muscle (*Dp427m*) isoform. IF and WB were performed using a patient quadricep muscle biopsy sample. Whole-genome sequencing was performed using blood-derived DNA. **a-c**: Performed by Boston Children's Hospital.

3.2 Evaluation of the functional of the regulatory element DME1

Patients with muscle exon 1 deletions, resulting in the absence of the dystrophin muscular isoform, are known not to develop DMD but instead X-linked dilated cardiomyopathy (XLDCM) [282], which is characterized by cardiac dysfunction without skeletal muscle involvement [283]. A question that arose was why Patient1 developed DMD.

Endogenous genetic rescue, in the form of up-regulating non-muscle dystrophin isoforms, has been observed in XLDCM patients with muscle isoform exon 1 (me1) deletion [282]. The full-length dystrophin protein (Dp427) has a molecular weight of 427 kDa. It has three isoforms, Dp427m, Dp427c, and Dp427p, transcribed from discrete promoters with distinct expression patterns. These isoforms are expressed in muscle, brain, and cerebellar Purkinje cells, respectively [284], and differ only in their promoter and exon 1 sequences from each other [138] (Fig. 1.2.3.2.1). The up-regulation of Dp427c and Dp427p in the muscle cells, in the absence of Dp427m, was indicated to be the reason why these exon-1 deletion patients developed XLDCM instead of DMD. This up-regulation was suggested to be associated with dystrophin muscle enhancer 1 (DME1), an enhancer element located closely downstream of me1 (DME1: GRCh38 chrX: 33,204,788-33,205,150; me1: GRCh38 chrX: 33,211,282-33,211,549). Previously, a promoter-luciferase reporter assay demonstrated that the DME1 element can enhance the activity of both the *Dp427c* promoter (GRCh38 chrX: 33,339,281-33,341,058) and the *Dp427p* promoter (GRCh38 chrX: 33,128,284-33,129,988) [282]. However, in

Patient1, both me1 and DME1 were removed by his mutation (Fig. 3.1.1d and Fig. 3.2.1), which may explain why Patient1 developed DMD. In fact, a previous study has reported that in a domestic cat patient, a deletion encompassing both *Dp427m* exon 1 and *Dp427p* exon 1 (and likely including the DME1 element between those two exon-1 regions) did not result in up-regulation of *Dp427c* within skeletal muscle, despite its intact sequence [285]. This observation aligns with our hypothesis concerning the pathology of Patient1.

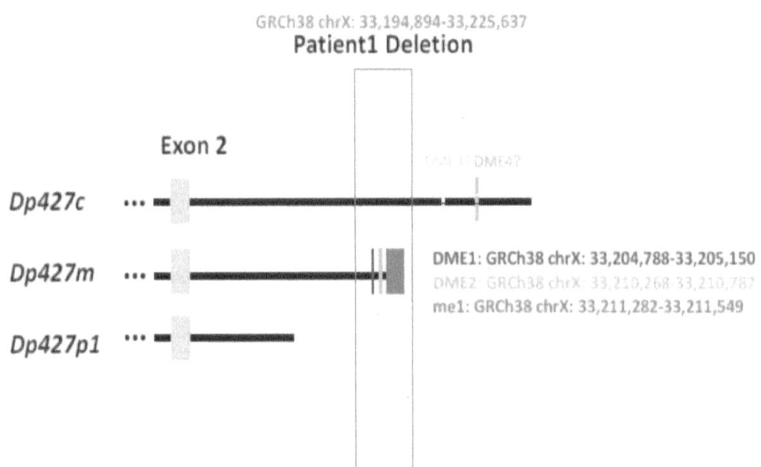

Fig. 3.2.1 Genomic locations of Patient1 deletion, DME1 and me1. Both me1 and DME1 were removed by Patient1 deletion. However, the deletion leaves the promoter and exon 1 of the cortical (*Dp427c*) and purkinje (*Dp427p*) isoforms of dystrophin intact.

To validate the *in situ* function of DME1, a lentiviral CRISPR-*Sa*Cas9 deletion experiment was designed. Two pairs of gRNAs were used to delete me1 and DME1, respectively, in the myoblast cell line 01UBIC (Fig. 3.2.2a,b). RNA was extracted from lentivirus-transduced pooled cells of each group and RT-qPCR was performed to evaluate the expression of *Dp427m* and *Dp427c*. The results showed that DME1 deletion reduced the expression level of *Dp427m* (Fig. 3.2.2c). me1 deletion increased the expression level of Dp427c. However, this overexpression was demolished when DME1 and me1 were both deleted (Fig. 3.2.2d). Together, these results indicated the existence of an endogenous genetic rescue mechanism in the myogenic cell line, involving the up-regulation of *Dp427c* in the absence of *Dp427m*. This up-regulation is likely regulated by DME1, but it may not be limited to DME1 since me1del-induced *Dp427c* up-regulation still occurred when DME1 was deleted (Fig. 3.2.2d: DME1&me1del *vs.* DEM1del, adjusted P-value=0.0039). Indeed, other enhancers that can regulate dystrophin expression in muscle tissues have also been reported, namely DME2, and potentially "DME3" and "DME4" [286,287]. In addition, many candidate enhancer elements have been identified by the Encyclopedia of DNA Elements (ENCODE) project, including EH38E2748907 (overlapping with DME1), EH38E2748908, EH38E2748910, EH38E2748911, and EH38E2748918, which are located in the same genomic region as me1, DME1, and DME2 [288]. These enhancers may also contribute to the me1del-induced *Dp427c* up-regulation. However, they were all absent in Patient1.

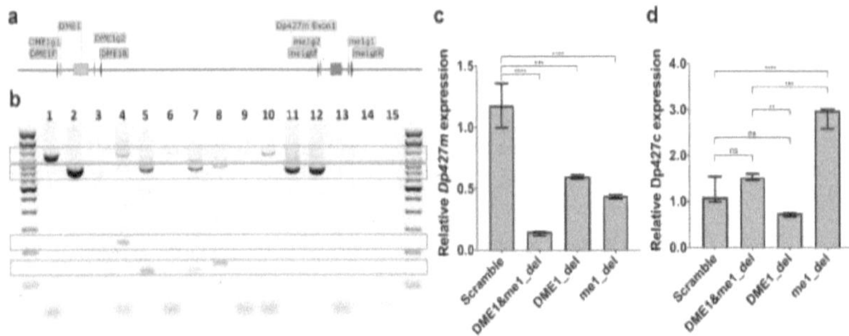

Fig. 3.2.2 DME1 is responsible for up-regulating *Dp427c* in the absence of *Dp427m*. a, The *Sa*Cas9 gRNA pairs used to make the deletions and the genotyping primers for the deletions. **b,** Genotyping for the samples. Blue rectangle: WT bands. Red rectangle: deletion bands. Lane1: Untreated cells; DME1 F+R; WT band 1114 bp. Lane2: Untreated cells; me1 F+R; WT band 854 bp. Lane3: Untreated cells; DME1 F+me1 R; WT product 7449 bp. Lane4: cells treated with DME1g1+g2; DME1 F+R; WT band 1114 bp; deletion band ~240 bp. Lane5: cells treated with me1g1+g2; me1 F+R; WT band 854 bp; deletion band ~133 bp. Lane6: cells treated with DME1g1+g2 and me1g1+g2; DME1 F+R; WT band 1114 bp; deletion band ~240 bp. Lane7: cells treated with DME1g1+g2 and me1g1+g2; me1 F+R; WT band 854 bp; deletion band ~133 bp. Lane8: cells treated with DME1g1+g2 and me1g1+g2; DME1 F+me1 R; WT band 7449 bp; deletion band ~155 bp. Lane9: cells treated with DME1g1; DME1 F+R; WT band 1114 bp. Lane10: cells treated with DME1g2; DME1 F+R; WT band 1114 bp. Lane11: cells treated with me1g1; me1 F+R; WT band 854 bp. Lane12: cells treated with me1g2; me1 F+R; WT band 854 bp. Lane13: Water; DME1 F+R. Lane14: Water; me1 F+R. Lane15: Water; DME1 F+me1 R. **c,d,** *Dp427m* (c) and *Dp427c* (d) expression in lentivirus-transduced pooled cells. DME1 deletion reduced the expression level of *Dp427m*. me1 deletion increased the expression level of *Dp427c*. However, this overexpression was demolished when DME1 and me1 were both deleted. To better control the experiment, the groups were balanced using the scramble lentivirus. Scramble: 4 units of the scramble lentivirus. DME1&me1_del: 1 unit of each of the four non-scramble lentiviruses. DME1_del: 2 units of the scramble lentivirus and 1 unit of each of the two DME1-targeting lentiviruses. me1_del: 2 units of the scramble lentivirus and 1 unit of each of the two me1-targeting lentiviruses. *GAPDH* was used as the housekeeping control for both *Dp427m* and *Dp427c*. Standard curves were made for *GAPDH*, *Dp427m* and *Dp427c* primers. Relative expression=*Dp427:GAPDH*. 3 biological replicates were set for each group. Median with 95% CI was indicated in the figures. Adjusted P-values: *P<0.0332; **P<0.0021; ***P<0.0002; ****P<0.0001 for the one-way ANOVA and Tukey's multiple comparison test. ns: nonsignificant.

Name	Purpose	Sequences (5'->3')
Scramble	Scramble gRNA	GGAGACGGACGTCTCT
DME1g1	gRNA1 for DME1 deletion	GCAAGGCAAAGAAGAATGAGGT
DME1g2	gRNA2 for DME1 deletion	GTTCTTAAGCACCAACATAAAA
me1g1	gRNA1 for me1 deletion	GTGTTCTGATTAATATCCAAAC

me1g2	gRNA2 for me1 deletion	GATTAACAAACCACTGCAGTAA
DME1F	Primer for DME1del genotyping	TTTCCACATTCAGAAACATTGC
DME1R	Primer for DME1del genotyping	AAGTGCTGACTTAAAGGGCAAG
me1gtf	Primer for me1del genotyping	TCTCACAGCAATCAAAATAAATCTG
me1gtr	Primer for me1del genotyping	TGCTTTTGTACTGAATAGTTTTTGTG
GAPDHF	qPCR primer for *GAPDH*	GAAGGTGAAGGTCGGAGTCA
GAPDHR	qPCR primer for *GAPDH*	TTGAGGTCAATGAAGGGGTC
Dp427mF	qPCR primer for *Dp427m*	TCTCATTGTTTTTAAGCCTA
Dp427R	qPCR primer for *Dp427m/Dp427c*	AAATTGTGCATTTACCCATTTTGTG
Dp427cF	qPCR primer for *Dp427c*	AGGAGAAAGATGCTGTTTTGCA

Table 3.2.3 gRNAs and primers used for DME1 and me1 deletion. Addgene plasmid 85452 was used as the backbone to clone the lentiviral *Sa*Cas9 constructs.

3.3 The rational design and the *in vitro* pre-clinical experiments of the CRISPRa construct

3.3.1 Endogenous genetic rescue

Although DME1 (and DME2) were both deleted in Patient1, we were still interested in investigating whether there was any extent of endogenous genetic rescue occurring in this patient. RNA was extracted from the patient's quadricep muscle biopsy sample by our collaborators in Dr. Louis Kunkel's lab and subsequently sent for RNA-seq. The RNA-seq indeed detected both *Dp427c* and *Dp427p* expression (Fig. 3.3.1.1), with *Dp427c* expression being higher than *Dp427p* (Fig. 3.3.1.1b and Table 3.3.1.2).

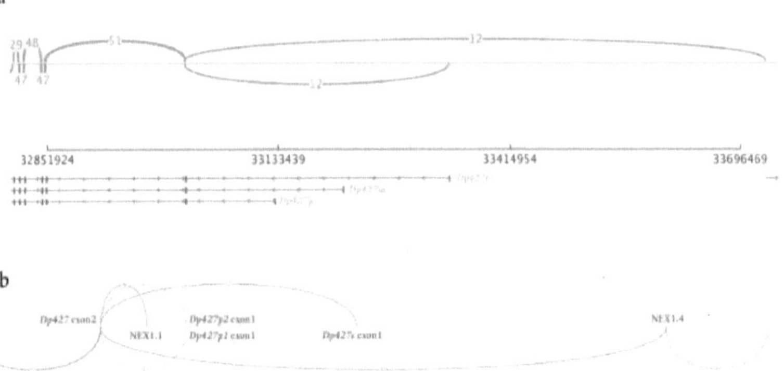

Fig. 3.3.1.1 Sashimi plot visualizing the RNA-seq results of Patient1 quadricep muscle biopsy. a, RNA-seq reads showing exons 1-7 (right to left) of the full-length *Dp427c* (cortical), *Dp427m* (muscle), and *Dp427p* (Purkinje) DMD isoforms (from top to bottom). The top panel displays the number of reads that span exons (arcs). Minimum junction coverage was set to 10 reads. The genomic coordinates are based on the GRCh38 reference genome. **b,** Sashimi plot depicting a different genomic window. Minimum junction coverage was set to 3 reads. NEX1.1: novel exon 1 region 1. NEX1.4: novel exon1 region 4. *Dp427p2* contains an additional 84 nucleotides directly after *Dp427p1* exon 1, resulting in the introduction of a stop codon 24 nucleotides downstream of the start codon [289].

Interestingly, aside from *Dp427c* and *Dp427p*, two types of novel isoforms were also identified, both of which share the same exon 2 as Dp427 (Fig. 3.3.1.1b). The exon preceding exon 2 in each novel isoform was labeled as "novel exon 1" or NEX1. NEX1 region1 (NEX1.1) (GRCh38 chrX: 33,078,186-33,078,302) overlaps with exon 2 (GRCh38 chrX: 33,078,186-33,078,347) of a previously identified transcript ENST00000682071.1 [290]. This "exon 2" is also annotated as the second exon of ENST00000683658.1 and was previously designated as DMD pseudoexon #04 (Fig. 3.3.1.5d and Fig. 3.4.1e) [291]. NEX1 region4 (NEX1.4) (GRCh38 chrX: 33,726,502-33,726,715) overlaps with a non-coding RNA gene (on the opposite strand) ENSG00000233928 (GRCh38 chrX: 33,726,337-34,346,527). The RNA-seq result suggested the presence of an additional exon upstream of NEX1.4 in some of the NEX1.4-containing transcripts (Fig. 3.3.1.1b).

In the NEX1.1-containing transcripts, situated within the same open reading frame (ORF) as *Dp427m* exon 2, the 38th codon preceding the first intact codon in exon 2 ("p.Glu12", p.Glu12 in Dp427m) is a methionine codon, which may serve as a start codon. However, the 30th codon before "p.Glu12" is a TGA stop codon (the 8th codon downstream of the potential start codon), suggesting that the NEX1.1-containing transcripts are unlikely to generate a full-length dystrophin. Nonetheless, these transcripts may still produce near-full-length dystrophin using downstream start codons (e.g., p.Met124 or p.Met128 in Dp427m), similar to the *Dp412e* isoform [292] and other isoforms identified in patients with certain mutations in *Dp427m* exon1-5 [293,294].

In the NEX1.4-containing transcripts, the 28th codon preceding the "p.Glu12" codon is a methionine codon. If this methionine codon serves as a start codon, it holds the potential to generate a full-length dystrophin with an N-terminal peptide "MAQLRGLQETPENAAEDGFTDVIKSRAD" preceding the "p.Glu12" residue.

Isoforms	GRCh38 coordinates (last 20 bases)	Total coverage (last 20 bases)
Dp427m	chrX:33211282-33211301	12
NEX1.1-containing	chrX:33078186-33078205	142
Dp427p1	chrX:33128147-33128166	73
Dp427c	chrX:33339259-33339278	244
NEX1.4-containing	chrX:33726502-33726521	576

Table 3.3.1.2 RNA-seq coverage of different exon 1 regions. The last 20 bases of each exon 1 region were used to examine the coverage.

Because of the high coverage of NEX1.4 in the RNA-seq result (Table 3.3.1.2), we became interested in identifying the transcription start site (TSS) of this novel isoform. First, we attempted to use RT-PCR to validate the existence of the transcript of this novel isoform (Table 3.3.1.3). We successfully validated the existence of NEX1.4 using RNA from Patient1 muscle biopsy (Fig. 3.3.1.4), but failed to detect it in two cell lines, Patient1-MyoD-converted-fibroblast (both in myoblast-like status and myotube-like status) and Patient1-iPSC-derived-myoblast.

Name	Sequence	Note
LONG_NEX1.4_F	TGCTGTGGAGAGCATCAAACGGACCGCACG	PCR validation of NEX1.4; expected band size 310 bp
LONG_exon3_R	GCCTTCGAGGAGGTCTAGGAGGCGCCTCCC	PCR validation of NEX1.4; expected band size 310 bp
HPRT1_F*	GGGGCCTGCTTCTCCTCAGCTTCAGGCGGC	*HPRT1* RT-PCR expected band 335 bp
HPRT1_R	CATCTCCTTCATCACATCTCGAGCAAGACG	*HPRT1* RT-PCR expected band 335 bp
LONG_exon3_Rnew	GGCGCCTCCCATCCTGTAGGTCACTGAAGA	5'RACE for NEX1.4

Table 3.3.1.3 Primers used to study NEX1.4. *The consensus TSS of *HPRT1* has been updated since the design of HPRT1_F. Hence, currently (Aug., 2023), the in-silico PCR tools may not be able to predict the product listed here.

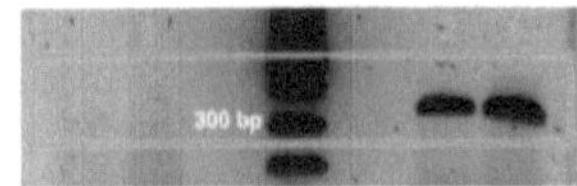

Fig. 3.3.1.4 RT-PCR validation of NEX1.4. Lane1: NEX1.4, RNA from Patient1 muscle biopsy. A faint band (~310 bp) can be observed in this lane. Lane2: NEX1.4, RNA from Patient1-MyoD-converted-fibroblast (Myotube-like status). Lane3: *HPRT1*, RNA from Patient1 muscle biopsy. Lane4: *HPRT1*, RNA from Patient1-MyoD-converted-fibroblast (Myotube-like status).

Next, we performed 5' Rapid Amplification of cDNA Ends (5' RACE) (Takara, 634858) and Topoisomerase-based cloning (TOPO cloning) (Invitrogen, 450159) using the RNA from Patient1 muscle biopsy to identify the TSS of NEX1.4 (Table 3.3.1.3). Two major bands, approximately 650 bp and 800 bp in size, were generated by 5' RACE (Fig. 3.3.1.5a-c). Sanger sequencing confirmed the presence of NEX1.4 sequence in the products within the 650-bp band (Fig. 3.3.1.5b), while the products in the 800-bp band likely originated from *Dp427c*, *Dp427p*, and other transcripts (Fig.

3.3.1.5c). For the 650-bp band, TOPO cloning was performed, and several colonies were selected for Sanger sequencing. The results revealed variable TSSs of NEX1.4-containing transcripts (Fig. 3.3.1.5g), with the most distant TSS localizing at GRCh38 chrX: 33,726,856. One out-of-frame upstream ORF (uORF) (GRCh38 chrX: 33,726,835-33,726,852) is observed in the 5' UTR of the longest NEX1.4-containing transcript, which may reduce the translation efficiency of the potential NEX1.4-specific dystrophin [295].

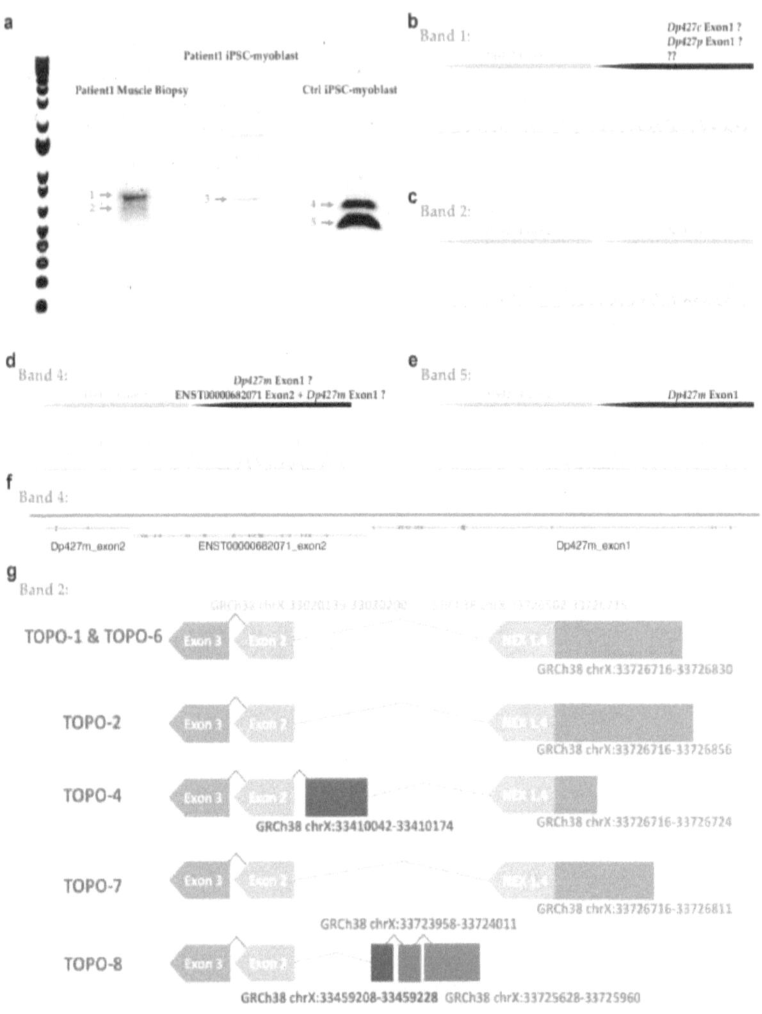

Fig. 3.3.1.5 5' RACE and TOPO cloning for the identification of NEX1.4 TSS. a, 5' RACE using RNA from Patient1 muscle biopsy, Patient1-iPSC-derived-myoblast, or Healthy-control-iPSC-derived-myoblast. Band 3 was a non-specific band, and its sequence was mapped to a gene called *TTC7B*. **b,** The Sanger sequencing result for Band 1 indicates that it may be a mixture of products amplified from *Dp427c*, *Dp427p*, and potentially other transcripts. **c,** The Sanger sequencing result for Band 2 indicates it is a mixture of different products, with a majority containing the NEX1.4 sequence. **d,** The Sanger sequencing result for Band 4 indicates it is a mixture of two types of products, with one amplified from *Dp427m* (or other transcripts that share the *Dp427m* exon 1-2 continuous region) and the other amplified from a group of non-canonical transcripts (like ENST00000682071 or ENST00000683658, f). **e,** The Sanger sequencing result for Band 5 indicates it is amplified from *Dp427m* (or other transcripts that share the

Dp427m exon 1-2 continuous region). g, TOPO cloning results for Band 2 reveal variable potential TSSs of transcripts containing the NEX1.4 sequence. TOPO-1, -2, -4, -6, -7, and -8 represent independent TOPO cloning colonies.

3.3.2 CRD-TMH-001 construct

Based on the preclinical assessments, we proposed to use gene therapy to enhance endogenous genetic rescue as a viable treatment for Patient1. For this strategy, three dystrophin isoforms were considered as candidate targets for up-regulation: Dp427c, Dp427p, and the potential NEX1.4-specific dystrophin. However, since there was insufficient evidence to conclusively demonstrate that NEX1.4-containing transcripts can generate a full-length dystrophin, the previously better-studied Dp427c and Dp427p were recognized as more favorable candidates. Additionally, the promoter of Dp427p can generate two different transcripts, *Dp427p1* and *Dp427p2*, with *Dp427p2* being unlikely to generate a full-length dystrophin [289]. Therefore, if we were to up-regulate the Dp427p promoter, a significant portion of the resulting transcripts would be nonfunctional (approximately half, estimated based on Fig. 3.3.1.1b). In this sense, Dp427c was presented as a more suitable candidate than Dp427p. As a side note, we did attempt to up-regulate *Dp427p*; however, no up-regulation was detected to the same extent as observed for *Dp427c* under similar conditions (Fig. 3.3.2.1a).

CRISPRa has been established as a viable option for achieving targeted gene up-regulation [296,297]. To customize a CRISPRa construct for Patient1, four crucial decisions needed to be made: firstly, selecting the suitable Cas protein; secondly, selecting the optimal gRNA sequence(s); thirdly, determining the appropriate promoters to drive the expression of the CRISPR-based construct; and fourthly, choosing the most suitable activator(s) to implement.

CRISPR-based gene therapy for muscle diseases currently relies on the use of AAV to deliver the construct. However, the maximum genome capacity of AAV is constrained to approximately 5 kb [54]. While many designs have employed two AAV vectors to deliver dual components [296,298] (Fig. 3.3.2.1h and Fig. 3.3.2.3d), such strategies may escalate manufacturing costs and engender concerns regarding efficacy and safety in clinical trials. These concerns arise from the necessity to administer at least double the total AAV dose to facilitate the functionality of the constructs (Fig. 3.3.2.4a-c). As a result, selecting a compact Cas protein that, along with the activator domains, can be accommodated within a single AAV vector is crucial for CRISPRa clinical applications. Recently, a growing variety of small-sized Cas proteins have emerged, including CasΦ [299] and CasMINI [300]. More recently, a eukaryotic programmable RNA-guided endonuclease, Fanzor, was identified, exhibiting an even smaller size (under 500 aa) [301]. However, during the time of treatment development for Patient1, such smaller nucleases were either unavailable or not sufficiently tested. Consequently, we opted for a relatively small Cas9, the one from *Staphylococcus aureus*, denoted as *Sa*Cas9 [302,303].

The efficiency of a particular gRNA in CRISPRa can be influenced by various factors, including but not limited to the gRNA sequence [304], the surrounding sequence context [305], and its distance from the TSS [306]. It is generally agreed that gRNAs targeting the region spanning -500 to -50 bp relative to the TSS tend to yield optimal gene up-regulation using CRISPRa [124,307-309]. However, given the potential for genes to exhibit variable TSSs [310-312], and the divergence in TSS annotations among different databases [306], an exclusive reliance on a solitary reported TSS may fail to offer a comprehensive depiction of the transcription initiation landscape. For example, the TSS of *Dp427c*, as reported in NM_000109.3, is situated at the -221 site in relation to the TSS indicated in NM_000109.4. Considering this significant variability, it may prove valuable to extend the search for the optimal gRNA to a broader window, such as -500 to +100 bp relative to a reported TSS.

Utilizing the gRNA design tool CHOPCHOP [313], a total of 8 gRNAs were designed and evaluated for up-regulating Dp427c. These gRNAs were denoted as C1 to C8 (Table 3.6.2). Among them, C7 consistently demonstrated high level of efficiency in various tests (Fig. 3.3.2.1b-e,g-l). Interestingly, we observed synergistic effects in several experiments when using multiple gRNAs simultaneously (Fig. 3.3.2.1c-f,h,j). However, due to safety considerations for clinical application, we refrained from employing a synergistic strategy in the treatment development for Patient1.

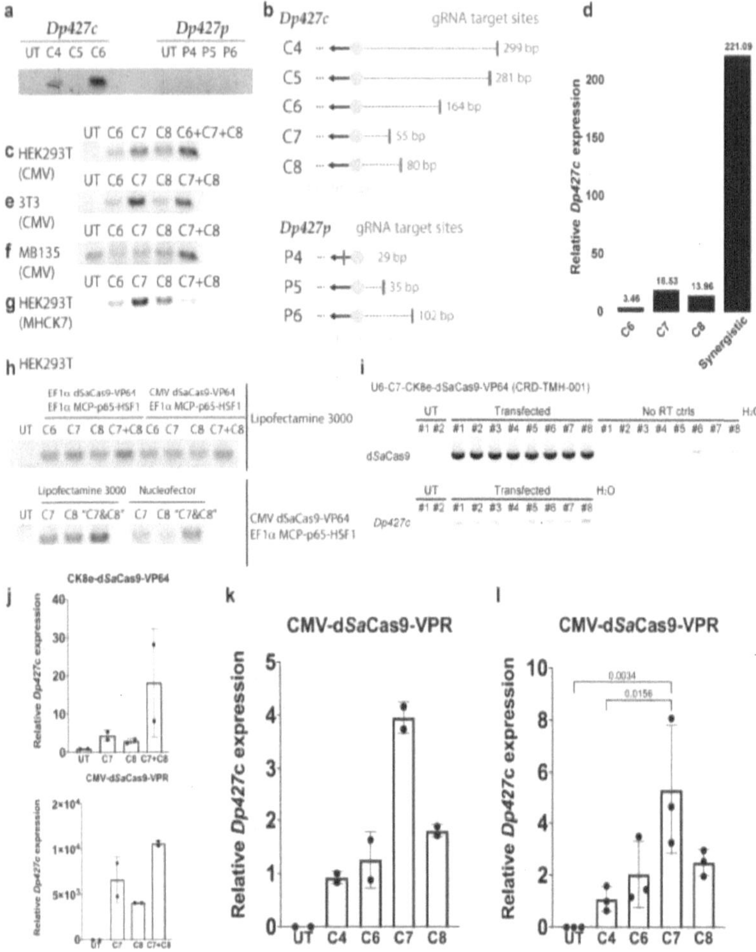

Fig. 3.3.2.1 C7 is the optimal gRNA for CRISPRa treatment for Patient1. a, Compared to *Dp427p*, *Dp427c* is a more suitable target for up-regulation. The constructs utilized in this experiment were based on the CMV-d*Sa*Cas9-VPR backbone and were introduced into HEK293T cells using Lipofectamine 3000. Sanger sequencing was performed to validate the bands. **b,** The distances between the gRNA target sites ("protospacer") and the TSSs. The distance is defined as the length of the region between the most 5' nt of the "protospacer" and the TSS. **c-h,** C7 exhibited optimal up-regulation in different experimental setups. Gel bands represent RT-PCR product of *Dp427c* **c,** The constructs utilized in this experiment were based on the CMV-d*Sa*Cas9-VPR-EF1α-BSD backbone and were introduced into HEK293T cells using Lipofectamine 3000. Blasticidin drug selection was performed to remove the untransfected cells. **d,** Same RNA samples as (c) were used for RT-qPCR. *GAPDH* was used as the housekeeping control. 3 qPCR triplicates were performed, and the mean Ct values were used to calculate the relative expression of *Dp427c*, 2^(*GAPDH*_Ct-*Dp427c*_Ct). Synergistic: C6+C7+C8. **e,** The constructs utilized in this experiment were

based on the CMV-d*Sa*Cas9-VPR-EF1α-BSD backbone and were introduced into 3T3 cells using Lipofectamine 3000. Blasticidin drug selection was performed. 3T3 is mouse embryonic fibroblast. Hence, mouse *Dp427c* primers were used. **f**, The constructs utilized in this experiment were based on the CMV-d*Sa*Cas9-VPR-EF1α-BSD backbone and were introduced into MB135 cells using Lipofectamine 3000. Blasticidin drug selection was performed. MB135 is a human myoblast healthy control. Baseline *Dp427c* expression was observed in the untransfected cells. **g**, The constructs utilized in this experiment were based on the MHCK7-d*Sa*Cas9-VPR-EF1α-BSD backbone and were introduced into HEK293T cells using Lipofectamine 3000. Blasticidin drug selection was performed to remove the untransfected cells. MHCK7 is a muscle specific promoter, yet we observed its leaky expression in HEK293T. **h**, Preliminary tests for the dual-vector systems. "C7&C8": two U6 cassettes were cloned into the same plasmid. PCR reactions using p65 primers were also performed as controls. **c,e-h**, PCR reactions using d*Sa*Cas9 primers were also performed as controls. C6+C7+C8: 1/3 amount of each plasmid was combined to test the synergistic effects. C7+C8: 1/2 amount of each plasmid was combined. **i**, The up-regulation driven by C7 is reproducible. 8 transfection replicates were performed in HEK293T using the U6-C7-CK8e-d*Sa*Cas9-VP64 (CRD-TMH-001) construct. 35 PCR cycles were performed. **j**, The synergistic effect of C7+C8 was primarily evaluated using qPCR (transfection duplicates were performed). The data were normalized to one UT sample. **k,l**, qPCR results confirmed C7 as the gRNA with the highest up-regulation among those tested. Transfection duplicates (k) or triplicates (l) were performed. The data were normalized to one C4 sample. **j-l**, Lipofectamine 3000 transfection in HEK293T. qPCR triplicates were performed. qPCR standard curves were generated for *Dp427c* and *GAPDH*. Relative *Dp427c* expression was *Dp427c*: *GAPDH* normalized to one of the samples. Plots depicted mean with SD. **l**, Adjusted p-values were generated using Tukey's multiple comparisons test. **a,c,e-l**, UT: untreated.

Selecting an appropriate promoter is also a key consideration in gene therapy [314]. Ideally, the chosen promoter should ensure expression at the desired level and specifically in the intended tissues [315]. The human U6 (hU6 or U6) promoter, an RNA polymerase III promoter recognized for its efficient expression of short RNAs, is a widely accepted choice for gRNA expression in CRISPR-related studies [316-318]. Furthermore, hU6 was employed in the first-ever CRISPR-based *in vivo* gene therapy clinical trial, EDIT-101 by Editas Medicine and Allergan, which was aimed at restoring vision loss in Leber congenital amaurosis type 10 (LCA10) [81,82]. In the treatment development for Patient1, we also utilized the hU6 promoter for the expression of the gRNAs. Notably, a study has reported that hU6 exhibits nucleosome redundancy, and its size can be significantly reduced by removing the non-functional region without decreasing the efficiency [319]. Indeed, in another project conducted in the Lek lab, we compared the efficiency of the U6 promoter (241 bp) with a minimized U6 (miniU6) promoter (103 bp), and no significant difference was observed. However, until now, there has been a lack of sufficient in vivo testing for the miniU6 construct, resulting in uncertainties regarding its efficacy and safety.

For the promoter of the dSaCas9-activator construct, the aim is to achieve strong expression in muscle tissues while minimizing expression in other tissues. Several muscle-specific promoters, including the muscle creatine kinase (MCK)-based promoters such as MHCK7 (770 bp, Fig. 3.3.2.1g) and CK8e (436 bp), have been established [320,321]. MHCK7 was utilized for the expression of a micro-dystrophin construct in SRP-9001, developed by Sarepta Therapeutics, the first FDA-approved gene therapy for DMD [322]. CK8e was employed in the clinical trial of another micro-dystrophin construct (SGT-001, NCT03368742) [323-325]. Considering its relatively compact size and previously reported robust muscle specificity [326], we chose CK8e for the development of the clinical construct for Patient1.

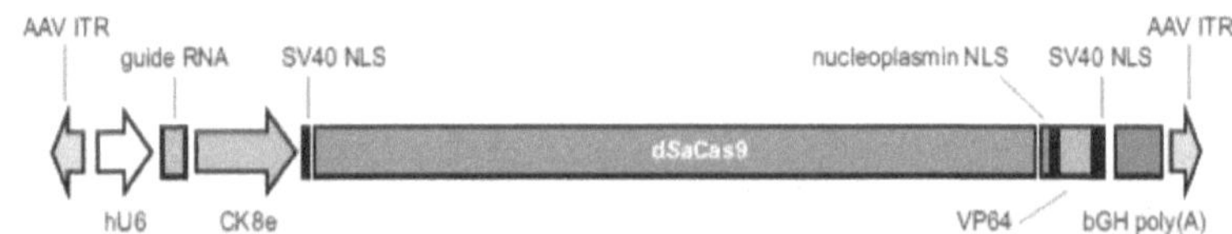

Fig. 3.3.2.2 The map of the U6-C7-CK8e-dSaCas9-VP64 (CRD-TMH-001) construct. The region between the ITRs measures 4558 bp in length.

Although various activators are available for use in CRISPRa, during the development of the treatment for Patient1, we could only design two systems that could fit into a single AAV vector: the single-VP64 system (Fig. 3.3.2.2) and the dual-VP64 system (Fig. 3.3.2.3a). The single-VP64 system has been utilized in pre-clinical CRISPRa experiments aimed at rescuing obesity caused by haploinsufficiency [327]. The dual-VP64 system has been utilized in pre-clinical experiments aimed at up-regulating *LAMA1* to compensate for mutations in *LAMA2*, which cause Merosin-deficient congenital muscular dystrophy (MDC1A) [296,297].

While the dual-VP64 system exhibited superior performance to the single-VP64 system in our *in vitro* experiments (Fig. 3.3.2.3b-e), it resulted in lower up-regulation in our *in vivo* experiments compared to the single-VP64 system (Fig. 3.3.2.4d-f). Our preliminary experiments indicated that there might have been rearrangement issues with the dual-VP64 system (Fig. 1.2.3.1.1 and Fig. 3.3.2.4g-i). From our initial findings, we could not determine the underlying essence or cause of the rearrangement that resulted in significantly weaker *in vivo* up-regulation than anticipated based on the *in vitro* experiment. The heterogeneity of the viral particle genome of the dual-VP64 system was assessed using native and alkaline gels, as per a protocol previously described [328], by our collaborators at UMass Medical School. Notably, no significant truncation was observed, implying that the rearrangement issue is more likely to occur post-transduction rather than during AAV manufacturing. Nonetheless, given the urgency of the treatment development for Patient1, we decided to proceed with the single-VP64 system for the pre-clinical experiments instead of attempting to further troubleshoot the dual-VP64 system.

As a side note, we designed and created three new dual-VP64 systems with different arrangements of elements, aiming to address the issues associated with the original system. Out of those three new systems, the one with the d*Sa*Cas9-VP64-VP64 arrangement order performed slightly better in terms of up-regulation level than the original system in *in vitro* experiments. Whether this arrangement order can solve the rearrangement issues needs further testing.

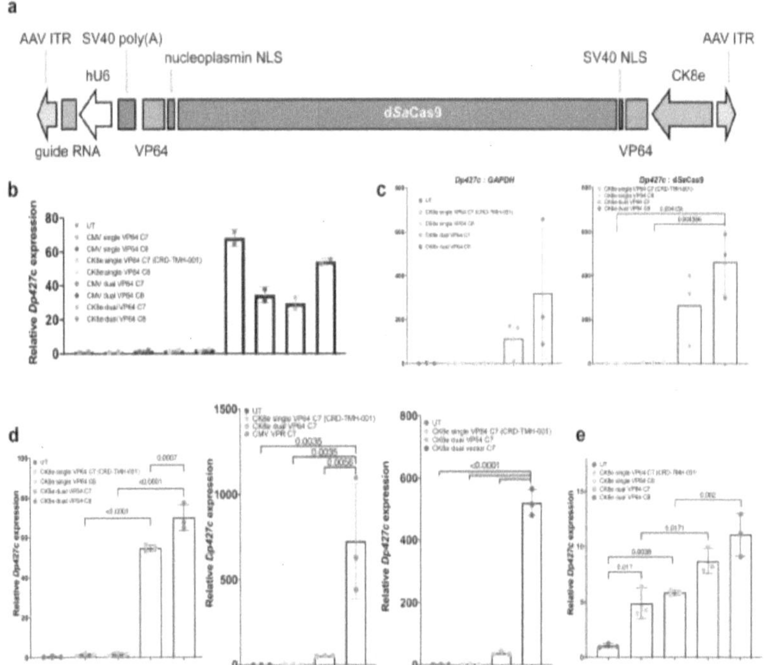

Fig. 3.3.2.3 *in vitro* experiments demonstrated the potential of other systems capable of achieving significantly higher up-regulation than the d*Sa*Cas9-VP64 system. a, The construct map of the CK8e-dual-VP64 system. The region between the ITRs measures 4566 bp in length. **b-e,** The dual-VP64 system can achieve a higher up-regulation than the single-VP64 system regardless of the promoter used. Interestingly, when employing the CK8e-dual-VP64 system, C8 exhibited better performance than C7. **b,** The data were normalized to one CMV-singleVP64-C7 sample (transfection replicate n=2). **d,** The VPR system (CMV-VPR-C7) and the dual-vector system (CK8e-d*Sa*Cas9-VP64 & U6-C7-U6-C8-MS2-CK8e-MCP-p65-HSF1) have the potential to achieve a substantially higher level of up-regulation compared to the VP64 systems. **c,d** The data were normalized to one CRD-TMH-001 sample (transfection replicate n=3). **e,** The data were normalized to one UT sample (transfection replicate n=3). **b-e,** Lipofectamine 3000 transfection in HEK293T (**b-d**) or MB135 myoblast (**e**). qPCR triplicates were performed. qPCR standard curves were generated for *Dp427c*, *GAPDH*, and d*Sa*Cas9. Relative *Dp427c*

expression was *Dp427c*: *GAPDH* normalized to one of the samples. Plots depicted mean with SD. Adjusted p-values were generated using Tukey's multiple comparisons test. UT: untreated.

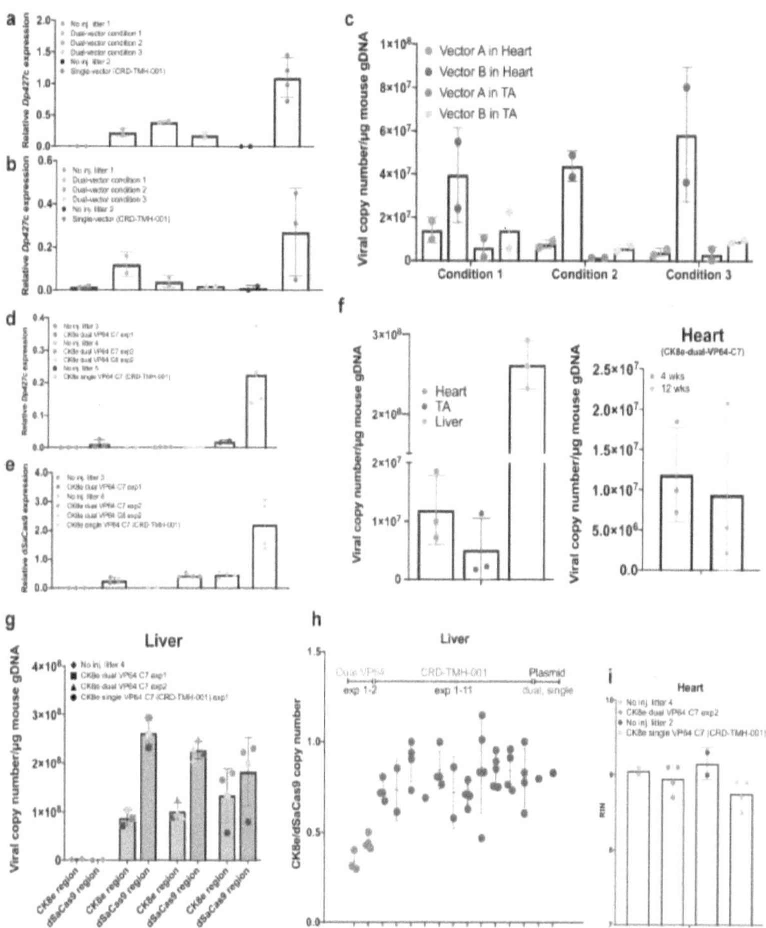

Fig. 3.3.2.4 ***in vivo*** **experiments using alternative systems demonstrated lower up-regulation in comparison to the single-VP64 system. a,b,** Even with stronger promoters, the dual-vector system achieved lower up-regulation compared to the single-vector system (**a**, Heart; **b**, TA: tibialis anterior). The dual-vector system was: CMV-dSaCas9-VP64 (Vector A) + U6-C7-U6-C8-MS2stemloop-EF1α-MCP(N55K)-p65-HSF1 (Vector B). Non-injected litter 1 (Mouse No. 20-38 & 20-39) and Non-injected litter 2 (Mouse No. 8365 & 8377) were the control groups for the dual-vector system and the single-vector system respectively. Condition 1: A, 2.1e14 vg/kg; B, 2.1e14 vg/kg (Mouse No. 20-42 & 20-43). Condition 2: A, 1.3e14 vg/kg; B, 2.6e14 vg/kg (Mouse No. 20-46 & 20-47). Condition 3: A, 6.1e13 vg/kg; B, 3.1e14 vg/kg (Mouse No. 20-50 & 20-51). Single-vector system: CRD-TMH-001, 2.8e14 vg/kg (Mouse No. 3009 to 3012; 3011 was excluded from the TA analysis due to non-specific

amplification as indicated by qPCR melting curve analysis). **c**, Viral copy numbers in samples utilizing the dual-vector system were comparable to those in samples utilizing the single-vector system. Samples from the same mice as in (**a**) and (**b**) were used. **a-c** Samples were collected 8 weeks after the AAV9 injection. **d,e**, The *in vivo* experiment results of the dual-VP64 system failed to replicate the strong up-regulation observed in the in vitro experiments. Non-injected litter 3 (Mouse.No. 20-84 to 20-86), Non-injected litter 4 (Mouse No. 21-12 & 21-13), and Non-injected litter 5 (Mouse No. 8339 & 8341) were the control groups for the dual-VP64 system exp1, dual-VP64 system exp2, and the single-VP64 system respectively. Dual-VP64 system exp1: CK8e-dual-VP64-C7, 1e14 vg/kg (Mouse No. 20-81 to 20-83). Dual-VP64 system exp2: CK8e-dual-VP64-C7, 2e14 vg/kg (Mouse No. 21-14 to 21-17); CK8e-dual-VP64-C8, 1.8e14 vg/kg (Mouse No. 21-18 to 21-21). Single-VP64-system: CRD-TMH-001, 2.8e14 vg/kg (Mouse No. 3005 to 3008). Samples were collected from heart tissues 4 weeks after the AAV9 injection. **f**, Viral copy numbers (quantified by d*Sa*Cas9 sequence) in samples utilizing the dual-VP64 system were comparable to those in samples utilizing the single-VP64 system. Samples were collected from: Mouse No. 20-81 to 20-83 (left; right, 4weeks) and Mouse No. 20-106 to 20-108 (1e14 vg/kg; right, 12 weeks). **g,h** Different regions of the viral genome in the dual-VP64 construct exhibited varying *in vivo* viral copy numbers, suggesting the occurrence of rearrangement or truncation events. Samples were collected from liver tissues. Non-injected litter 4: Mouse No. 21-12 & 21-13. Dual-VP64 experiments were with the CK8e-dual-VP64-C7 construct. Dual-VP64 exp1 (4 weeks post injection): Mouse No. 20-81 to 20-83. Dual-VP64 exp2 (4 weeks post injection): Mouse No. 21-14 to 21-17. Single-VP64 experiments were with the CRD-TMH-001 construct. Single-VP64 exp1 (8 weeks): 2.8e14 vg/kg, Mouse No. 3009 to 3012. Single-VP64 exp2 (4 weeks): 2.8e14 vg/kg, Mouse No. 21-24 & 21-25. Single-VP64 exp3 (4 weeks): 2e14 vg/kg, Mouse No. 21-26 to 21-29. Single-VP64 exp4 (8 weeks): 2.8e14 vg/kg, Mouse No. 21-62. Single-VP64 exp5 (8 weeks): 2e14 vg/kg, Mouse No. 21-63 to 21-66. Single-VP64 exp6 (6 months): 2e14 vg/kg, Mouse No.21-103 & 21-104. Single-VP64 exp7 (6 months): 2e14 vg/kg, Mouse No. 21-108 to 21-112. Single-VP64 exp8 (4 weeks): 2e13 vg/kg, Mouse No. 2021 to 2025. Single-VP64 exp9 (4 weeks): 4e13 vg/kg, Mouse No. 3021 to 3025. Single-VP64 exp10 (4 weeks): 2.2e14 vg/kg, Mouse No. 21-214 to 21-217. Single-VP64 exp11 (4 weeks): 2.5e14 vg/kg, Mouse No. 2203 to 2206. **g**, Data points with the same color represent the same mouse for a given construct. **h**, The CK8e dual VP64 plasmid and the CRD-TMH-001 plasmid were included in the qPCR as references. **a-h**, qPCR triplicates were performed. qPCR standard curves were generated for *hDp427c*, *mHprt1*, d*Sa*Cas9 cDNA, d*Sa*Cas9 sequence, WPRE sequence, CK8e sequence, and mdx sequence. Relative *Dp427c* expression was *hDp427c*: *mHprt1*. Relative d*Sa*Cas9 expression was d*Sa*Cas9 (cDNA): *mHprt1*. Vector A copy number was quantified using the d*Sa*Cas9 standard curve. Vector B copy number was quantified using the WPRE standard curve. Input mouse genome DNA (gDNA) was quantified using the mdx standard curve. Plots depicted mean with SD. **i**, RNA Integrity Number (RIN) was measured for a subset of the samples, all of which displayed high RIN values, indicating that the observations were not a result of poor RNA quality. Non-injected litter 4: Mouse No. 21-12 & 21-13. Dual-VP64 exp2 (4 weeks post injection): Mouse No. 21-14 to 21-17. Non-injected litter 2: Mouse No. 8365 & 8377. Single-VP64 (8 weeks post injection): Mouse No. 3009 to 3012. **a-i**, The viral doses were computed based on the quantifications provided by the manufacturers.

Considering all these factors within the development process, we concluded by choosing the U6-C7-CK8e-d*Sa*Cas9-VP64 construct for implementation in both the pre-clinical experiments and the clinical trial for Patient1. This construct was subsequently designated as CRD-TMH-001 during the FDA Investigational New Drug (IND) application and the clinical trial phase.

3.3.3 *in vitro* evaluation of the effects of the on- and off-target CRISPRa up-regulation

Because VP64 alone is not the most potent activator, in our *in vitro* experiments with CRD-TMH-001, *Dp427c* up-regulation can only be consistently observed in the HEK293T cell line, and the up-regulation level is weak (Fig. 3.3.2.1i,j and Fig. 3.3.2.3b-d). The up-regulation induced by CRD-TMH-001 was not consistently reproducible in other cell lines, although occasional instances of up-regulation were detected in MB135 cells (Fig. 3.3.2.3e).

Regarding the on- and off-target effects, our primary focus revolved around two aspects: firstly, examining the on-target effects on the transcriptome stemming from the up-regulation of *Dp427c*; secondly, investigating off-target effects leading to the up-regulation of other genes. These effects were either the result of gRNA binding to sites with mismatches or gRNA-independent binding driven by the activator. We argued that due to the inability of the CRD-TMH-001 construct to induce detectable up-regulation in Patient1-specific cell lines and its limited up-regulation level in HEK293T cells (Fig. 3.3.3.2a), it might not be effective for the intended evaluations. As a result, we decided to utilize the U6-C7-CMV-d*Sa*Cas9-VPR construct for these evaluations (Fig. 3.3.3.1a). Our rationale encompasses the following aspects: Firstly, this alternative construct can effectively induce *Dp427c* up-regulation in a Patient1-specific cell line (Fig. 3.3.3.2d,e), thus providing evaluations that are more contextually relevant. Secondly, it encompasses both the gRNA C7 and the activator VP64, making the off-target effects observed with this construct not entirely irrelevant to CRD-TMH-001. Furthermore, the inclusion of more activators increases the likelihood of detecting off-target up-regulation within the transcriptome.

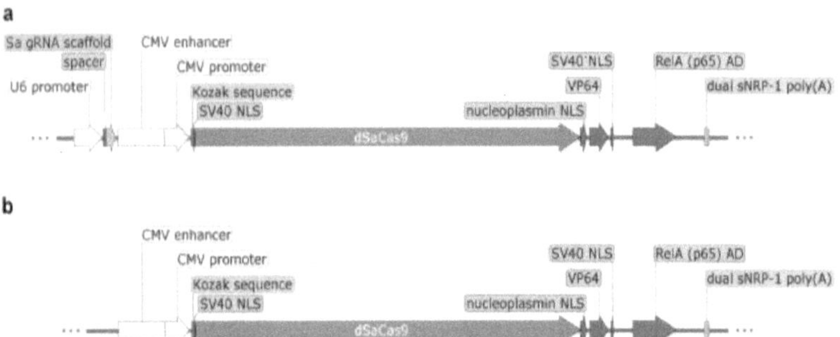

Fig. 3.3.3.1 Plasmid maps of the CMV-dSaCas9-VPR system. a, The construct with the U6-C7 cassette. **b,** The VPR-only construct.

Targeted qPCRs were conducted to evaluate the up-regulation effects on both the intended target and potential off-target genes. In addition to *Dp427c*, we specifically focused on another three genes that are likely associated with off-target effects and may have oncogenic implications: *KIAA1217* [329], *SSX2IP* [330], and *UGGT1* [331] (Table 3.3.3.3). We did not observe up-regulation of these potential off-target genes in either HEK293T (Fig. 3.3.3.2a-c) or Patient1 iPSC-derived myoblast (iSMS) cells (Fig. 3.3.3.2d,e). While we did observe down-regulation of the off-target genes in Patient1 iSMS (Fig. 3.3.3.2d), we believed that this down-regulation might have been a consequence of utilizing the inappropriate control (untransfected, UT) in this context. Indeed, upon employing the VPR-only transfection control, the observed down-regulation was eliminated (Fig. 3.3.3.2e). We also observed up-regulation of *KIAA1217* in an experiment conducted using MB135 myoblasts (Fig. 3.3.3.2f). Nevertheless, considering the peculiarly higher expression of d*Sa*Cas9 in the VPR-only control compared to the C7 group, coupled with the substantially lower on-target up-regulation compared to other cell lines, we proposed that this observation is specific to MB135 and may not hold significant clinical implications regarding off-target effects.

Next, we conducted RNA-seq analysis to evaluate the on- and off-target effects across the entire transcriptome. To enhance the likelihood of detecting meaningful signals, we employed the CMV-VPR system (U6-C7-CMV-d*Sa*Cas9-VPR *vs.* CMV-d*Sa*Cas9-VPR) in HEK293T cells (Fig. 3.3.3.1 and Fig. 3.3.3.2h-j). The RNA-seq was conducted on the NovaSeq 6000 platform, yielding approximately 70 M to 100 M reads per sample. The RNA-seq analysis captured the expression of the C7 gRNA (Fig. 3.3.3.2h) and a subtle signal of *Dp427c* up-regulation (Fig. 3.3.3.2i and Table 3.3.3.4). However, the evidence is inadequate to definitively ascertain the existence of functional up-regulation. Given the weak on-target up-regulation signal, we argue that RNA-seq might lack the sensitivity to detect potential off-target up-regulation events.

The RNA-seq analysis generated a list of differentially expressed genes (absolute log2(fold change)>=0.5, adjusted p-value<0.1) (Table 3.3.3.4), yet elucidating the factors contributing to their altered expression is complex. Potential explanations encompass downstream effects of *Dp427c* up-regulation, cellular responses to the expression of the C7 gRNA, as well as off-target up-regulation and its subsequent downstream effects. Nevertheless, none of the differentially expressed genes are among the predicted C7 off-target site-associated genes (Table 3.3.3.3 and Table 3.3.3.4).

The TissueEnrich analysis [332] indicated that the differentially expressed genes exhibit some enrichment in muscle tissues (Fig. 3.3.3.2k). However, the GeneMANIA [333] analysis did not yield any predictions regarding genetic or physical interactions among the differentially expressed genes and *DMD*, though it did reveal co-expression, co-localization, and shared protein domains among certain genes (Fig. 3.3.3.2l). Furthermore, the top hit gene *SMIM11* [log2 (fold change)=-3.74, adjusted p-value=7.85e-79] appears to be a previously understudied gene, and consequently, our literature review did not yield much information about this gene.

Genes that were up-regulated and might pose a high oncogenic risk (OncoScore >30 [334]) include: *FAM117A* [335,336], *ID1* [337-339], *HOXB6* [340-342], *LLGL2* [343-346], *BMF* [347], *HOTAIR* [348,349], and *HCFC1R1* [350]. While our literature review did not uncover extensive cancer-related research on *HCFC1R1* (OncoScore=71.80), we did come across a preprint suggesting that HCFC1R1 might be involved in transporting HSV-1 VP16 into the nucleus [351]. It is worth highlighting that VP16 is the fundamental component of VP64.

Genes that were down-regulated and have an OncoScore >30 include: *INHBA* [352-354], *GEM* [355,356], and *TNFRSF12A* [357,358]. In addition, up-regulation of *Inhba* has been observed in a DMD mouse model (mdx/mTR) [359], while up-regulation of *Tnfrsf12a* has been observed in mdx mice [360].

FLNC was down-regulated in the C7 treated samples [log2 (fold change)=-0.53, adjusted p-value=5.39e-05]. Notably, it has been reported that in DMD patients, there is a significant increase in the amount of FLNc at the sarcolemma [361].

With those being discussed, it is crucial to recognize that these *in vitro* experiments can only provide a limited scope of insight. Hence, it remains challenging to definitively determine the consequences and implications of these differentially expressed genes, particularly concerning the clinical application of d*Sa*Cas9-based up-regulation. To obtain a more comprehensive understanding, further investigations into on- and off-target effects should be conducted in an *in vivo* setting.

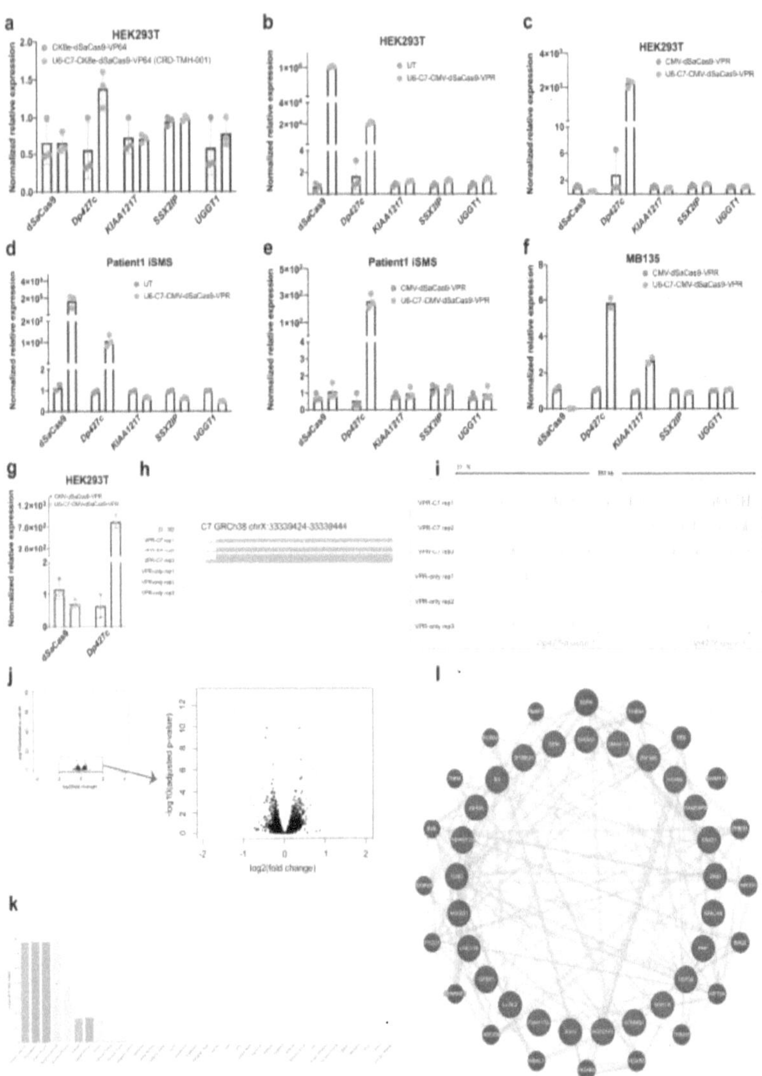

Fig. 3.3.3.2 ***in vitro*** **evaluation of the effects of the on- and off-target CRISPRa up-regulation. a,** CRD-TMH-001 generates modest *Dp427c* up-regulation in HEK293T cells. The data were normalized to one VP64-only control. **b-e,** In *in vitro* experiments, the U6-C7-CMV-d*Sa*Cas9-VPR construct exhibits strong *Dp427c* up-regulation. **b,d,** The data were normalized to one UT control. **c,e-g,** The data were normalized to one VPR-only control. **d,e,** iSMS: iPSC-derived myoblast. **a-g,** Lipofectamine 3000 transfection was performed. qPCR triplicates were performed. *GAPDH* (**a-f**) or *HPRT1* (**g**) was used as the housekeeping control. The relative expression was determined using: 2^(Ct_housekeeping_gene - Ct_gene_of_interest). **h-l,** RNA-seq was performed to evaluate the on- and off-target effects across the entire transcriptome. The RNA samples were from the same samples in (c) (transfection replicates n=3). The FASTQ files from

RNA-seq were aligned to the GRCh38 reference genome with STAR [362], and expression levels per gene were assessed with RSEM [363]. **h**, RNA-seq detected the C7 gRNA expression. These signals should be removed when evaluating the up-regulation of *DMD*. i, A higher read count was observed in the VPR-C7 samples within the region spanning from *Dp427c* exon 1 to *Dp427m* exon 1. However, most of the reads fell within the intronic region, making it difficult to conclusively determine whether functional up-regulation occurred based solely on this result. j, To perform differential gene expression analysis, the data was processed with DESeq2 [364], and differentially expressed genes were identified as genes with an absolute log2(Fold Change) of at least 0.5 and adjusted p-value of below 0.1 (Table 3.3.3.4). **k**, The differentially expressed genes exhibited some enrichment in muscle tissue. This figure was generated with TissueEnrich [332]. **l**, Co-expression, co-localization and shared protein domains were predicted by GeneMANIA among the differentially expressed genes and *DMD* [333].

Gene	Mismatch positions	Off-target "PAM"	GRCh38 coordinates	Type	OncoScore
KIAA1217	atgatgggaaagaggagctga	gagaat (valid)	chr10:24308167-24308193	Intronic	48.93
SSX2IP	atcatgtgaaatggcaactgt	gtggat (valid)	chr1:84652039-84652065	Intronic	48.59
UGGT1	agcacacgcaaggggagctgt	gggagg (weak)	chr2:128077784-128077810	Intergenic	30.75

Table 3.3.3.3 Potential off-target sites of the C7 guide RNA. A list of potential off-target sites was generated using CRISPOR [86]. Red: mismatched nts. Off-target "PAM" denotes the 6-nt sequence positioned adjacent to the 3' end of the gRNA off-target sites. Genes exhibiting a high OncoScore were selected for targeted qPCR evaluation. For reference, *TP53* holds an OncoScore of 90.61 [334]. NNGRRG is a less effective PAM sequence for SaCas9 [365]. Other potential off-target site-associated genes predicted by CRISPOR include: *VEPH1*, *TMEM54*, *ANKRD46*, *ACTN2*, and *AL031602*.

Gene	Gene name	log2 (fold change)	Adjusted p-value	OncoScore
ENSG00000205670.10	SMIM11	-3.741671778	7.85E-79	n/a
ENSG00000122641.10	INHBA	-1.206404417	2.26E-12	34.828351
ENSG00000076826.9	CAMSAP3	0.917283132	8.55E-11	17.454664
ENSG00000185437.13	SH3BGR	-0.859332946	2.67E-07	28.209315
ENSG00000180730.4	SHISA2	0.682605307	7.36E-07	26.333945
ENSG00000165698.15	SPACA9	0.793394593	2.29E-06	0
ENSG00000128591.15	FLNC	-0.532444746	5.39E-05	21.943676
ENSG00000109103.11	UNC119	0.523303133	0.000488639	11.647600
ENSG00000152137.6	HSPB8	-0.828014818	0.000551233	28.424449
ENSG00000121104.7	FAM117A	0.639530601	0.002015393	37.500000
ENSG00000148677.6	ANKRD1	-0.750010677	0.002015393	24.658689
ENSG00000125968.8	ID1	0.547907072	0.003335859	49.980276
ENSG00000164949.7	GEM	-0.525833217	0.005013302	35.022799
ENSG00000108511.9	HOXB6	0.515809379	0.005695703	37.665053
ENSG00000115461.4	IGFBP5	0.518795099	0.018471051	26.253001
ENSG00000166963.12	MAP1A	0.503973346	0.019837553	19.894164
ENSG00000115267.5	IFIH1	-0.644548849	0.019919936	16.456174
ENSG00000073350.13	LLGL2	0.519614248	0.024920108	58.751292
ENSG00000135643.4	KCNMB4	0.531187475	0.037198287	6.841231
ENSG00000104081.13	BMF	0.504079817	0.046123358	38.716306
ENSG00000124104.18	SNX21	0.506047635	0.047785158	27.591121
ENSG00000081665.13	ZNF506	-0.555555562	0.048862639	25.000000
ENSG00000228630.5	HOTAIR	0.560539623	0.053776053	58.382507
ENSG00000103145.10	HCFC1R1	0.504538946	0.057963554	71.795489
ENSG00000006327.13	TNFRSF12A	-0.654762554	0.058507774	77.421788

ENSG00000107201.9	RIGI	-0.620207685	0.096276225	23.826108
ENSG00000198947.15	**DMD***	**0.22632339**	**0.27179814**	n/a

Table 3.3.3.4 Differentially expressed genes between the VPR-C7 and VPR-only samples. To perform differential gene expression analysis, the data was processed with DESeq2 [364], and differentially expressed genes were identified as genes with an absolute log2(Fold Change) of at least 0.5 and adjusted p-value of below 0.1. None of these genes are present among the CRISPOR-predicted genes. *DMD* was included as a reference (*C7 reads excluded).

As a supplementary note, we also conducted additional *in vitro* evaluations. We developed a RT-(q)PCR workflow employing a primer pair targeting *Dp427* exon 23-24 to quantify the expression of *Dp427* (*Dp427c*, *Dp427m*, and *Dp427p*) (Fig. 3.3.3.5a). This primer pair was also utilized in another ongoing project within the lab, aiming to employ CRISPRa to upregulate *Dp427* for the treatment of BMD. This primer pair facilitated a direct comparison between gRNAs targeting the *Dp427c* promoter and those targeting the *Dp427m* promoters.

We also conducted a preliminary time-course experiment in Patient1 iPSC-derived myoblasts (Fig. 3.3.3.5b). Considering that lipofectamine transfection typically results in transient intracellular plasmid presence, the *Dp427c* signal detected after d*Sa*Cas9 ceased to express (Cas9 protein can be rapidly degraded in cells [366]) is hypothesized by us to stem from a remnant effect caused by the genomic accessibility change induced by the activator [126]. This hypothesis is particularly intriguing to us, as it suggests the potential for *Dp427c* up-regulation to persist even after the AAV has dissipated in the body over time. However, it's essential to note that this is a preliminary experiment, and further validation through well-designed experiments is warranted in both *in vitro* and *in vivo* settings.

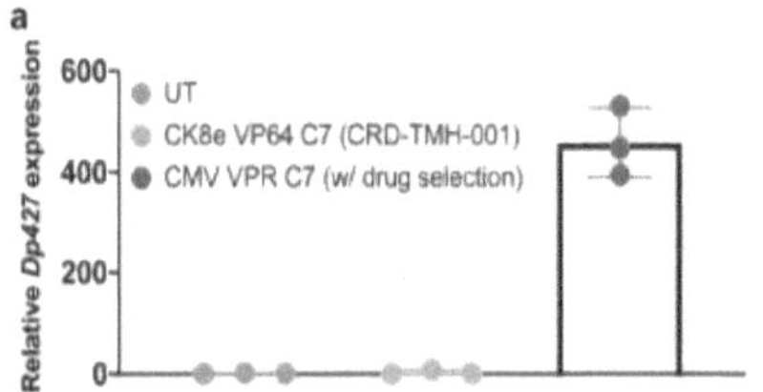

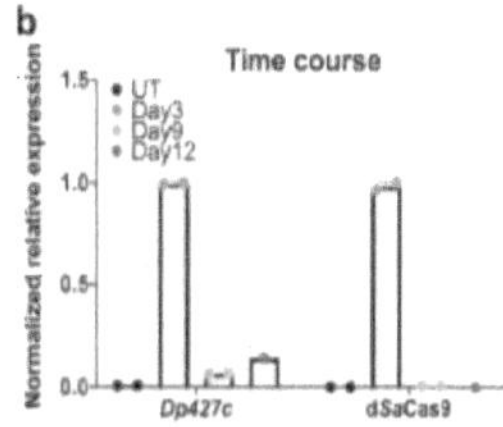

Fig. 3.3.3.5 Additional experiments for CRISPRa up-regulation evaluation. **A**, Establishing exon 23-24 qPCR for inclusive evaluation of *Dp427* transcripts (*Dp427m*, *Dp427c*, and *Dp427p*). The data were normalized to one CRD-TMH-001 sample (HEK293T, transfection replicate n=3). **B**, Preliminary time-course results suggest that the up-regulation might exhibit a remnant effect, even when dSaCas9 expression is no longer present. Additional validations are needed to make convincing conclusions. The data were normalized to one Day-3 sample (Patient1 iPSC-derived myoblast, Lipofectamine 3000 transfection, U6-C7-CMV-dSaCas9-VPR). **A,b**, qPCR triplicates were performed. qPCR standard curves were generated for *Dp427*, *Dp427c*, d*Sa*Cas9, and *GAPDH*. Relative *Dp427* expression was *Dp427*: *GAPDH* normalized to one of the samples. Relative *Dp427c* expression was normalized *Dp427c*: *GAPDH*. Relative d*Sa*Cas9 expression was normalized d*Sa*Cas9: *GAPDH*. Plots depicted mean with SD. UT: untreated.

3.4 *in vivo* pre-clinical experiments in the hDMD/mdxD2 mouse model

In our *in vivo* experiments, AAV was delivered into the mice through intravenous (IV) injections. Since the mouse strain we used was a humanized hDMD/mdxD2 strain (mdx: a nonsense mutation in exon 23 of *mDmd*; D2: DBA/2J genetic background, which generates more severe muscular dystrophy symptoms; 3.6), our initial task was to establish an RT-(q)PCR workflow that could precisely distinguish *hDp427c* from *hDp427m*, *mDp427c*, and *mDp427m*. A previous study had designed primers for this purpose [367], and when we tested those primers, they also exhibited good species/isoform specificity in our experiments (Fig. 3.4.1a-c).

We further optimized the qPCR conditions for the *hDp427c* primers to quantify *hDp427c* up-regulation (Fig. 3.4.1c and Table 3.6.4). It is important to note that the *hDp427c* primers can also capture an additional transcript, carrying a pseudoexon [291] (GRCh38 chrX: 33,078,186-33,078,347), which naturally occurs in *DMD* expression and is not a result of our experimental procedure (Fig. 3.4.1e). This pseudoexon-carrying transcript is positioned between exon 1 and exon 2, making it challenging to avoid in PCRs. While this may slightly complicate qPCR result interpretation, the expression of this transcript is closely linked to *Dp427c* expression, maintaining a linear relationship where up-regulation leads to a stronger signal.

At the meantime, we developed workflows utilizing C7 primers to quantify gRNA expression (Fig. 3.4.1f). Furthermore, we established workflows employing d*Sa*Cas9 primers to measure viral copy number and mdx primers to measure genome DNA input, enabling the evaluation of AAV biodistribution (Fig. 3.4.1d).

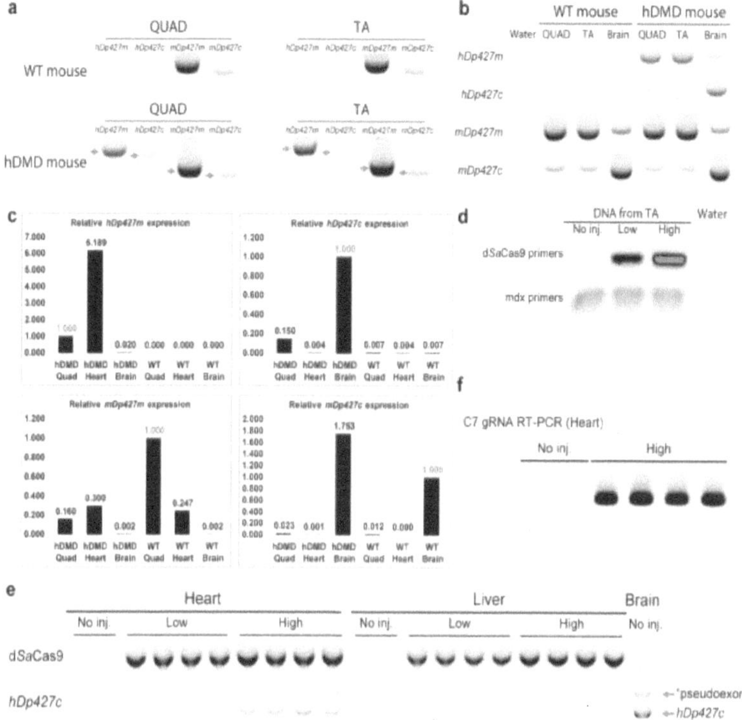

Fig. 3.4.1 Testing primers and optimizing experiment conditions required for different evaluations. a-c, The primers utilized in a previous study [367] also demonstrate high specificity in distinguishing transcripts of different isoforms in both mice and humans within our RT-PCR experimental context. Sanger sequencing confirmed the identity of the observed bands. hDMD mouse: RNA samples were extracted from a female hDMD/mdxD2 mouse (Mouse No. 20-05; homozygous for mdxD2 background and heterozygous for hDMD transgenic insertion). QUAD: quadricep. TA: tibialis anterior. 32 cycles (**a**) or 28 cycles (**b**) were performed for the PCR reactions. **c**, *Hprt1* was used as the housekeeping control. 3 qPCR triplicates were performed, and the mean Ct values were used to calculate the relative expression. RT-PCR was also performed and showed the same pattern. For the hDMD/mdxD2 samples, the qPCR was also repeated by another operator, which showed the same pattern. Red: the samples that were used for normalization. **d**, mdx primers (p9427 and p259E) can be employed to quantify DNA input, allowing for normalization of viral copy numbers in different tissues following AAV injection. No inj.: non-injected hDMD/mdx2 mouse (Mouse No. 8339). Low: a hDMD/mdxD2 mouse injected with 2.8e13 vg/kg CRD-TMH-001 AAV9 (Mouse No. 3002). High: a hDMD/mdxD2 mouse injected with 2.8e14 vg/kg CRD-TMH-001 AAV9 (Mouse No. 3008). The samples were collected four weeks after the injection. Red: saturated pixels. **e**, The d*Sa*Cas9 primers were employed to evaluate the expression of the Cas9 construct and The *hDp427c* primers were employed to evaluate the up-regulation. The *hDp427c* primers can generate 2 bands, with the major band being *hDp427c* (366 bp) and the minor band having a larger size. Sanger sequencing confirmed that the larger band had a pseudoexon (GRCh38 chrX: 33,078,186-33,078,347; pseudoexon #04 [291]) between *hDp427c* exon1 and exon2. Heart & liver samples were collected four weeks after the injection. No inj.: Mouse No. 8339 and 8341 (left to right). Low: CRD-TMH-001, 2.8e13 vg/kg, Mouse No. 3001-3004 (left to right). High: CRD-TMH-001, 2.8e14 vg/kg, Mouse No. 3005-3008 (left to right). The brain sample was collected from Mouse No. 20-05. **f**, Primers (v1) for RT-PCR for C7 gRNA

were primarily tested. No inj.: Mouse No. 8339 and 8341 (left to right). High: Samples were collected 8 weeks after the injection; CRD-TMH-001, 2.8e14 vg/kg, Mouse No. 3009-3012 (left to right).

In our pre-clinical experiments using hDMD/mdxD2 mice, our results consistently demonstrated that liver tissues exhibited the highest level of AAV9 biodistribution, followed by heart tissues (Fig. 3.4.2b,h, Fig. 3.4.3a, and Fig. 3.4.5a,d-f). The viral copy number decreased over time in the body. At the 6-month post-injection time point, the levels dropped to approximately 30% to 10% of the levels observed at the 4-week time point in heart, gastrocnemius (GA), and liver tissues (Fig. 3.4.2h).

For CK8e-driven d*Sa*Cas9-VP64 expression, the heart consistently exhibited the highest level of expression, followed by the skeletal muscle tissues (Fig. 3.4.2 a,c,e, Fig. 3.4.4b, and Fig. 3.4.5g). Notably, robust d*Sa*Cas9 expression was not observed in liver tissues, despite their high biodistribution (Fig. 3.4.2c and Fig. 3.4.5g). This indicated that CK8e indeed exhibited good muscle specificity and performed as anticipated in our experiments. Both CK8e-driven d*Sa*Cas9 and U6-driven C7 expression persisted at 6 months post injection. No significant changes in expression levels were observed when comparing the 4-week and 6-month time points for d*Sa*Cas9 and C7 in heart tissues (Fig. 3.4.2d,e). Western blot experiments were also conducted in our lab, confirming the presence of d*Sa*Cas9 protein expression, and the results were consistent with the qPCR findings.

The up-regulation of *hDp427c* was also most robust in the heart tissues, followed by the skeletal muscle tissues (Fig. 3.4.2 a,c,f,g and Fig. 3.4.5c,h). While the up-regulation could be consistently detected in heart tissues at the 4-week post-injection time point, it typically manifested in skeletal muscle tissues after 8 weeks post-injection

(Fig. 3.4.2a,f). While the *Dp427c* up-regulation could persist for a minimum of 6 months in heart tissues, its level might reduce to as low as approximately ~1/5 of the level observed at the 4-week time point (Fig. 3.4.2g). More carefully designed time-course experiments are needed and will be conducted in our follow-up studies to establish a deeper understanding of how the up-regulation persists in the body. The changes in *Dp427c* up-regulation over time could result from a complex interplay of factors, including AAV uncoating [368], viral copy loss [369], evolving CRISPRa intracellular efficacy [370], and possible genomic accessibility shifts [126].

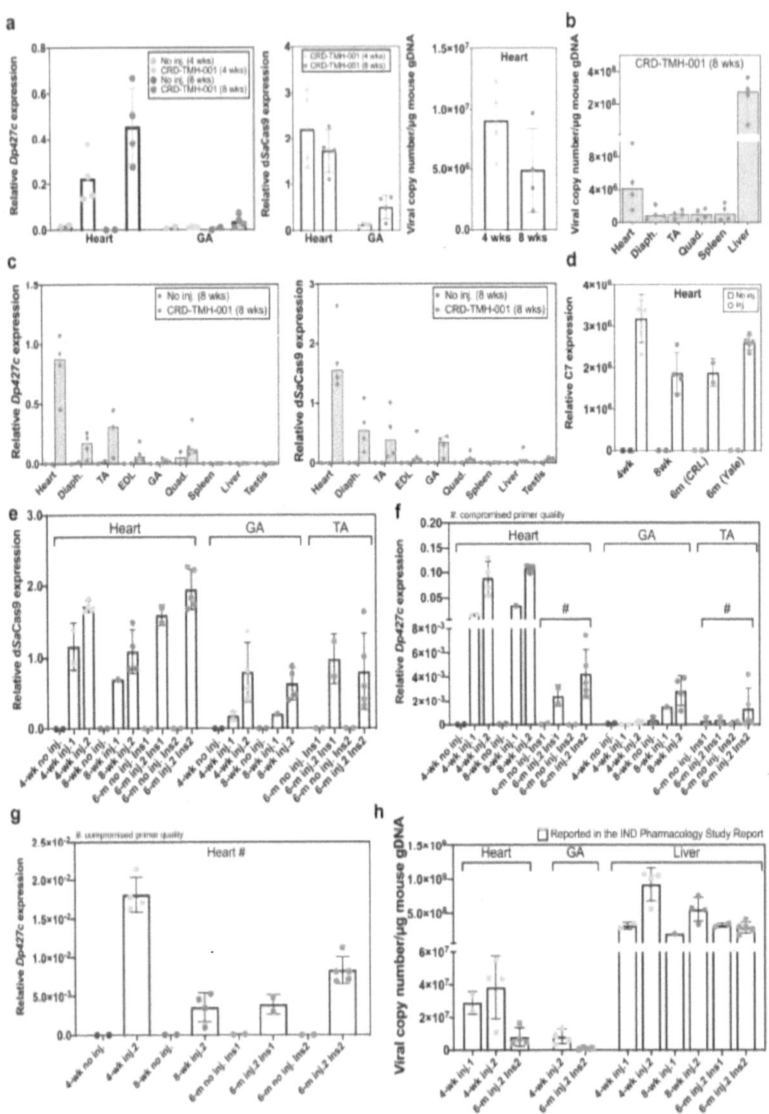

Fig. 3.4.2 Multiple independent injection experiments were conducted to evaluate *Dp427c* up-regulation, d*Sa*Cas9 expression, and AAV biodistribution. a, *Dp427c* up-regulation was detected in the heart at 4 weeks post-injection, and in the GA muscle at 8 weeks. **b,** Biodistribution analysis revealed that liver exhibited the highest AAV9 distribution. Heart was the second highest among the tissues tested. **c,** The highest levels of *Dp427c* up-regulation and d*Sa*Cas9 expression were observed in the heart tissue at 8 weeks. Data from the TA of mouse 3011 were excluded from the *Dp427c* analysis. **a-c,** AAV-injected Mice (Mouse No. 3005 to 3008), along with the non-injected control mice (Mouse No. 8339 & 8341), were

sacrificed 4 weeks post injection (CRD-TMH-001, 2.8e14 vg/kg). AAV-injected Mice (Mouse No. 3009 to 3012), along with the non-injected control mice (Mouse No. 8365 & 8377), were sacrificed 8 weeks post injection (CRD-TMH-001, 2.8e14 vg/kg). **d,e**, The expression of the CRISPRa system can persist for up to at least 6 months. **d**, C7 gRNA, qPCRs were run for all samples in the same batch. **e**, d*Sa*Cas9, qPCRs were run for the samples in batches following the exact same protocol. **f,g** The up-regulation of *Dp427c* can also persist for up to at least 6 months (Heart & TA). **f**, Peculiarly, in heart, despite the lack of significant changes in the expression levels of C7 (**d**) and d*Sa*Cas9 (**e**), the *Dp427c* up-regulation, although still detectable, displayed a substantial reduction at the 6-month time point. Later, we discovered that this discrepancy was likely caused by compromised *hDp427c* primer quality at the 6-month time point. **g**, the up-regulation at the 6-month time point was found to be more comparable to the other two time points, when we re-ran all the samples together using the same batch of primers. Notably, the same 4-wk and 8-wk samples as mentioned in (**f**), exhibited considerably lower signals compared to the results presented in (**f**). The data presented in (**e**) were generated concurrently with the data in (**f**). Given that the RNA quality seemed satisfactory in (**e**), we deduced that the significant reduction observed in (**f**) was likely due to the compromised quality of the *hDp427c* primers. Upon identifying this issue, we optimized our protocol for storing the primers. This is IMPORTANT for any pre-clinical experiment that necessitates a long study duration. **h**, the viral copy numbers at 6 months were approximately 3 to 8-fold smaller compared to those at the 4-week time point. **d-h**, CRD-TMH-001 AAV-injected Mice (Mouse No. 21-24 & 21-25, 2.8e14 vg/kg*; Mouse No. 21-26 to 21-29, 2e14 vg/kg#), along with the non-injected control mice (Mouse No. 21-22 & 21-23), were sacrificed 4 weeks post injection. CRD-TMH-001 AAV-injected Mice (Mouse No. 21-62, 2.8e14 vg/kg*; Mouse No. 21-63 to 21-66, 2e14 vg/kg#), along with the non-injected control mice (Mouse No. 21-60 & 21-61), were sacrificed 8 weeks post injection. CRD-TMH-001 AAV-injected Mice (Mouse No. 21-103 & 21-104), along with the non-injected control mice (Mouse No. 21-101 & 21-102), were sacrificed 6 months post injection (2e14 vg/kg#) (Kept at Charles River Laboratories, CRL, Ins1).CRD-TMH-001 AAV-injected Mice (Mouse No. 21-108 to 21-112), along with the non-injected control mice (Mouse No. 21-105 & 21-106), were sacrificed 6 months post injection (2e14 vg/kg#) (Kept at Yale, Ins2). *: Inj.1, This batch of AAV was stored at -80 °C for approximately one year. #: Inj.2. Mouse No. 21-110 was not used in the biodistribution analysis for heart and GA. **a-h**, No inj.: non-injected mice. Inj.: injected mice. GA: gastrocnemius. Diaph.: diaphragm. TA: tibialis anterior. EDL: extensor digitorum longus. Quad.: quadriceps. 4wk: 4 weeks. 8wk: 8 weeks. 6m: 6 months. qPCR triplicates were performed. Relative *Dp427c* expression was *hDp427c* : *mHprt1*. Relative d*Sa*Cas9 expression was d*Sa*Cas9 (cDNA) : *mHprt1*. Relative C7 expression was C7 : *mHprt1*.Viral biodistribution was quantified with d*Sa*Cas9 sequence and mdx sequence standard curves. Plots depicted mean with SD. qPCR standard curves: *hDp427c* (standard curve 1), *mHprt1* (standard curve 1), d*Sa*Cas9 cDNA (standard curve 1), dSaCas9 sequence (standard curve 1), mdx sequence (standard curve 1), and C7 version 1 (standard curve 1) (Table 3.6.5).

Dose-response effects were observed, demonstrating a correlation between increased dosages and higher levels of d*Sa*Cas9-VP64 expression, which led to greater up-regulation of *Dp427c* (Fig. 3.4.2e,f,h, Fig. 3.4.3, and Fig. 3.4.5d-h). For the evaluation of the Good Manufacturing Practice (GMP) batch of CRD-TMH-001 AAV9 intended for the clinical trial, we investigated both high (2e14 vg/kg) and low (1e14 vg/kg) doses of the substance in hDMD/mdxD2 mice. The biodistribution, d*Sa*Cas9 expression, and *Dp427c* up-regulation matched our expectations, in line with prior results (Fig. 3.4.5d-h). Furthermore, toxicity studies were performed at Charles River Laboratories (Study No. 01559002), and no adverse events were observed. Taking into account Patient1's low lean muscle mass of 45%, our extensive team decided to employ the 1e14 vg/kg dose for the clinical trial.

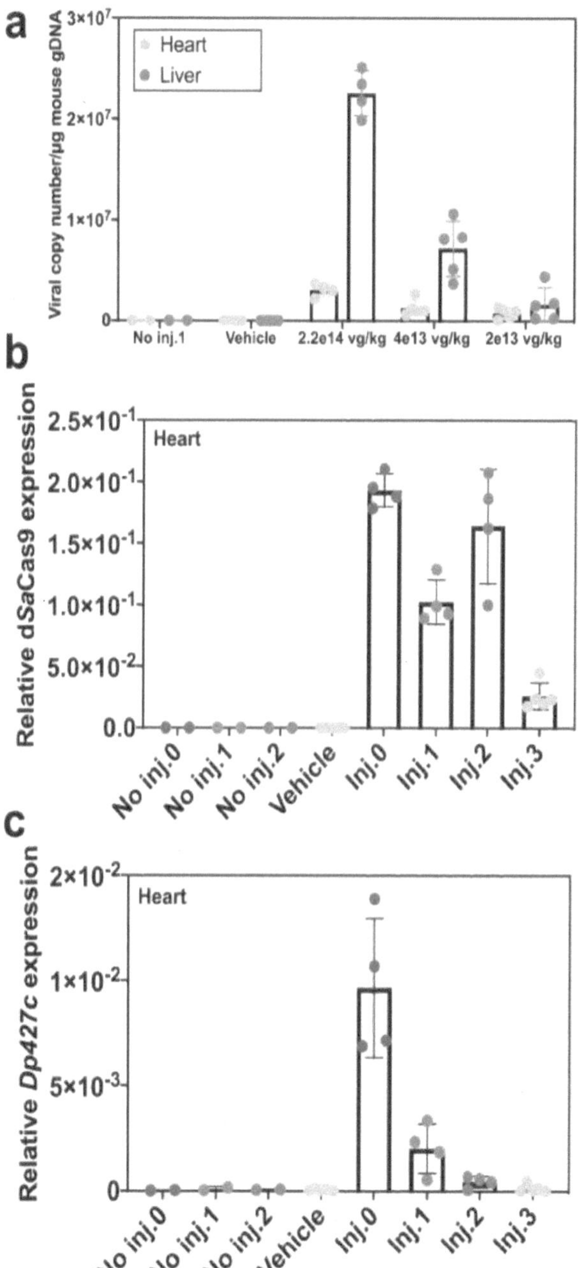
a
Viral copy number/µg mouse gDNA
3×10^7
2×10^7
1×10^7
0
Heart
Liver
No inj.1
Vehicle
2.2e14 vg/kg
4e13 vg/kg
2e13 vg/kg
b
Relative dSaCas9 expression
2.5×10^-1
2.0×10^-1
1.5×10^-1
1.0×10^-1
5.0×10^-2
0.0
Heart
No inj.0
No inj.1
No inj.2
Vehicle
Inj.0
Inj.1
Inj.2
Inj.3
c
Relative Dp427c expression
2×10^-2
1×10^-2
5×10^-3
0
Heart
No inj.0
No inj.1
No inj.2
Vehicle
Inj.0
Inj.1
Inj.2
Inj.3

Fig. 3.4.3 Intravenous injections in hDMD/mdxD2 mice using the CRD-TMH-001 GMP AAV9 manufactured by Viralgen. a-c, The up-regulation of *Dp427c* exhibited a dose-response effect, where higher doses of AAV result in greater up-regulation. **a,** Mice used to test Viralgen GMP AAV9: Mouse No. 1021 to 1025 were vehicle injected controls. Mouse No. 2021 to 2025 were treated with CRD-TMH-001 at a lower dose (2e13 vg/kg) and Mouse No. 3021 to 3025 were treated at a relatively higher dose (Inj.3, 4e13 vg/kg). Mouse No. 21-212 & 21-213 were non-injected controls (No inj.1). Mouse No. 21-214 to 21-217 were treated with CRD-TMH-001 at a high dose (Inj.1, 2.2e14 vg/kg). Samples were collected 4 weeks post injection. **b,c** 4-week post-injection heart RNA from Mouse No. 21-26 to 21-29 (Inj.0, CRD-TMH-001, 2e14 vg/kg reported, 4.6e14 vg/kg Viralgen re-titered), along with the non-injected control mice Mouse No. 21-22 & 21-23 (No inj.0), and Mouse No. 3005 to 3008 (Inj.2, CRD-TMH-001, 2.8e14 vg/kg reported, 7e13 vg/kg Viralgen re-titered), along with the non-injected control mice Mouse No. 8339 & 8341 (No inj.2) were utilized to synthesize cDNA and perform qPCR in a same batch as the RNA samples from the mice used to test the Viralgen GMP, ensuring a fair comparison. **a-c,** qPCR triplicates were performed. Relative *Dp427c* expression was *hDp427c* : *mHprt1*. Relative d*Sa*Cas9 expression was d*Sa*Cas9 (cDNA) : *mHprt1*. Viral biodistribution was quantified with d*Sa*Cas9 sequence and mdx sequence standard curves. Plots depicted mean with SD. qPCR standard curves: *hDp427c* (standard curve 2), *mHprt1* (standard curve 2), d*Sa*Cas9 cDNA (standard curve 2), dSaCas9 sequence (standard curve 2), and mdx sequence (standard curve 2) (Table 3.6.5). Upon completing this set of experiments, it became evident that the yield of the GMP AAV9 manufactured by Viralgen was inadequate for the intended clinical trial.

A major concern in utilizing AAV for delivering CRISPR-based constructs is the potential for on-site genomic integration [85]. The use of the dead *Sa*Cas9 system theoretically eliminates the likelihood of such a scenario. However, to take additional precautions, we examined the potential occurrence of undesired on-site integration after administering CRD-TMH-001. No instances of on-site integration or indels were observed in the livers or hearts of mice injected with CRD-TMH-001 at the 6-month post-injection time point (Fig. 3.4.4).

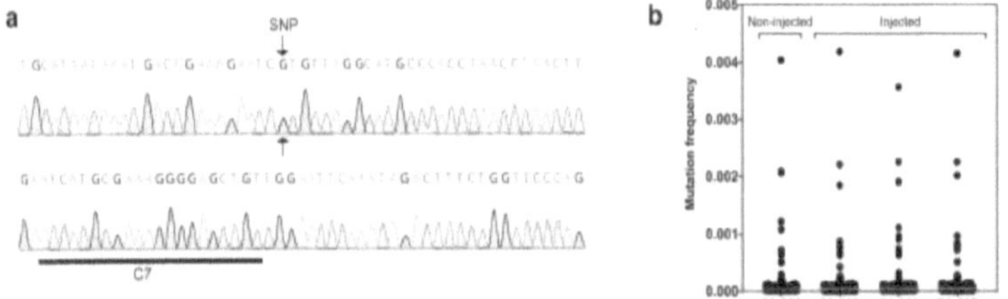

Fig. 3.4.4 No on-site indels or integration events were detected. a, No C7 CRISPRa-related genomic changes were detected by Sanger sequencing [liver & heart DNA from Mouse No. 21-108, 21-109, 21-

111, and 21-112 (CRD-TMH-001, 2e14 vg/kg, 6 months post injection); heart DNA from Mouse No. 21-105 (non-injected)]; though interestingly, we identified a single nucleotide polymorphism (SNP) in the hDMD/mdxD2 mice used for the study (GRCh38 chrX: 33339475 T->C, Global minor allele frequency: 0.01669). Figure depicts Sanger sequencing result of the PCR product utilizing liver DNA from Mouse No. 21-112 as the template. **b**, No significant mutations were identified by NGS in the injected mice compared to the non-injected mice. Liver DNA samples were utilized as templates. For each site within the region GECh38 chrX:33339330-33339471, the read frequency of each nucleotide distinct from the reference genome was computed. Red lines: median.

While the FDA issued a "Safe to Proceed" letter for our IND application, there remain numerous unresolved issues that necessitate attention for research purposes. During the development of CRD-TMH-001, our top priority was preparing for the n-of-1 clinical trial and meeting the requirements set forth by the FDA. However, our experiments were somewhat inadequate in fully establishing the efficacy of CRD-TMH-001. This deficiency, with full awareness by Patient1, his family, the entire extensive team, and the FDA, is evident in the following aspects: first, while we consistently detected the d*Sa*Cas9 protein using western blot, we have yet to establish a method to ensure elevated levels of the Dp427c protein; second, we were unable to assess physiological improvement following the administration of CRD-TMH-001. Both challenges arose from the use of hDMD/mdxD2 mice, which are fundamentally healthy, instead of a Patient1-specific model mouse strain. Recently, our collaborators and we have obtained a novel mouse strain that can mimic the Patient1 mutation (hDMD_muscle_exon1_del/mdxD2). We plan to address the aforementioned issues while also evaluating potential adverse events using this strain as a more context-appropriate model.

Another issue to address in our *in vivo* experiments is that the d*Sa*Cas9-VP64 C7 RNP complex can also target the C7 genomic site in *mDmd* in mice due to the conservation of C7 across evolution and its identical sequence in both humans and mice (GRCm38 chrX: 82814839-82814859). Despite the presence of the mdx mutation (ENSMUST00000114000 chrX:g.83803333C>T; c.2983C>T; p.Q995*) in *mDmd* in mdx mice, this unintended targeting might still lead to issues such as unwanted competition between the human and mouse C7 genomic sites, and potential up-regulation of certain isoforms of mouse *Dmd*. These possible scenarios warrant careful consideration, and if necessary, removal of the C7 genomic site from the *mDmd* locus.

A significant challenge we encountered during our development process is the variability in AAV titering due to the use of different quantification methods by different manufacturers (Fig. 3.4.3). For the improvement of the AAV gene therapy field, it's crucial to establish a standardized quantification method [371-373].

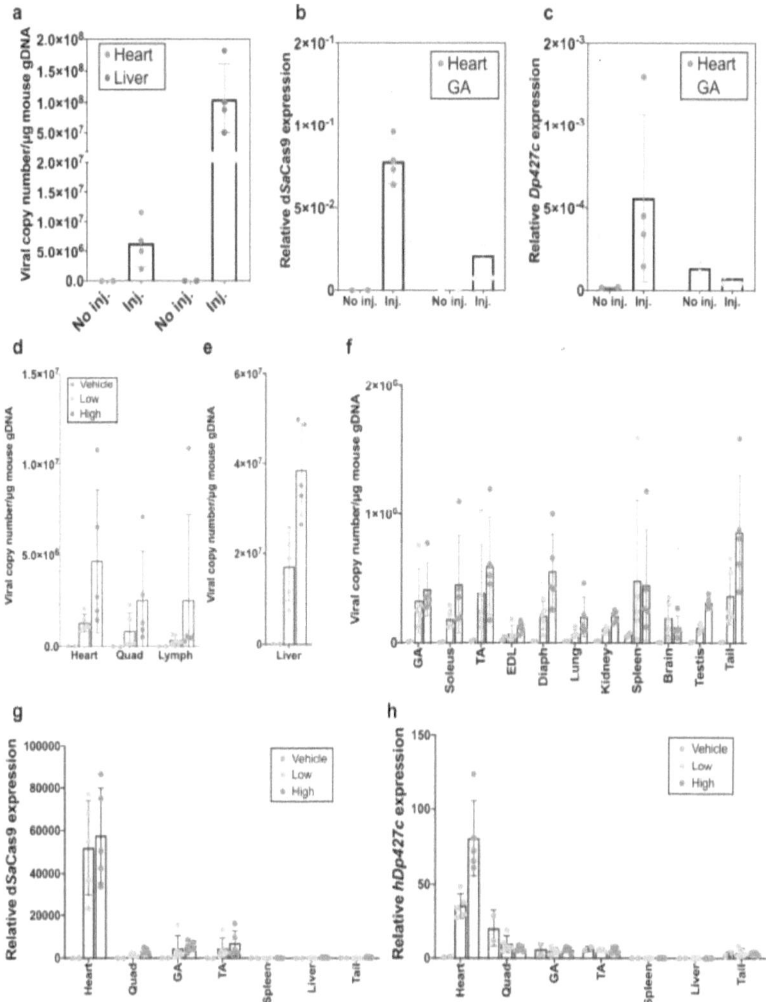

Fig. 3.4.5 Intravenous injections in hDMD/mdxD2 mice using the CRD-TMH-001 Research-grade and GMP AAV9 manufactured by Andelyn. a-c, Andelyn research-grade AAV9 demonstrated expected biodistribution (**a**), d*Sa*Cas9 expression (**b**), and *hDp427c* up-regulation (**c**). Mice used to test Andelyn research-grade AAV9: Mouse No. 2201 & 2202 were non-injected control. Mouse No. 2203 to 2206 were treated with 2.5e14 vg/kg CRD-TMH-001. Samples were collected 4 weeks post injection. **d-h,** Andelyn GMP AAV9 demonstrated expected biodistribution (**d-f**), d*Sa*Cas9 expression (**g**), and *hDp427c* up-regulation (**h**). No adverse events were observed. Mice used to test Andelyn GMP AAV9: Mouse No. Tox1011 & Tox1012 were vehicle-injected control. Mouse No. Tox2011 to Tox2015 were treated with 1e14 vg/kg CRD-TMH-001 (low). Mouse No. Tox3011 to Tox3015 were treated with 2e14 vg/kg CRD-TMH-001 (high). Samples were collected 4 weeks post injection. **d-f,** AAV9 exhibited the highest level of biodistribution in the liver (**e**), followed by the heart and Quad (**d**). There was an outlier mouse in

the lymph node tissue group. However, the biodistribution in the lymph nodes was otherwise not notably high. **g**, Heart tissues exhibited the highest level of d*Sa*Cas9 expression, followed by the skeletal muscle tissues. **h**, At the 4-week time point, robust up-regulation of *Dp427c* was only detected in heart tissues. **a,d-f**,: qPCR standard curves: d*Sa*Cas9 sequence (standard curve 2) and mdx sequence (standard curve 2) (Table 3.6.5). **b,c**, qPCR standard curves: *hDp427c* (standard curve 2), *mHprt1* (standard curve 2), and d*Sa*Cas9 cDNA (standard curve 2) (Table 3.6.5). **g,h**, qPCR standard curves: *hDp427c* (standard curve 3), *mHprt1* (standard curve 3), and d*Sa*Cas9 cDNA (standard curve 3) (Table 3.6.5). **a-h**, qPCR triplicates were performed. Relative *Dp427c* expression was *hDp427c* : *mHprt1*. Relative d*Sa*Cas9 expression was d*Sa*Cas9 (cDNA) : *mHprt1*. Viral biodistribution was quantified with d*Sa*Cas9 sequence and mdx sequence standard curves. Plots depicted mean with SD. No inj.: non-injected. Inj.: injected. GA: gastrocnemius. Quad: quadriceps. Lymph: lymph nodes. TA: tibialis anterior. EDL: extensor digitorum longus. Diaph: diaphragm.

In our pre-clinical experiments, we observed that lymph node tissues (mandibular, mesenteric, and popliteal lymph node tissues placed in a single tube) showed notably varied results in both biodistribution (Fig. 3.4.5d) and gene expression (Fig. 3.4.6). We speculated that this variability could originate from the uneven distribution of AAV within lymph node tissues [374,375]. This highlights the necessity for an improved protocol when collecting lymph node tissues in future studies.

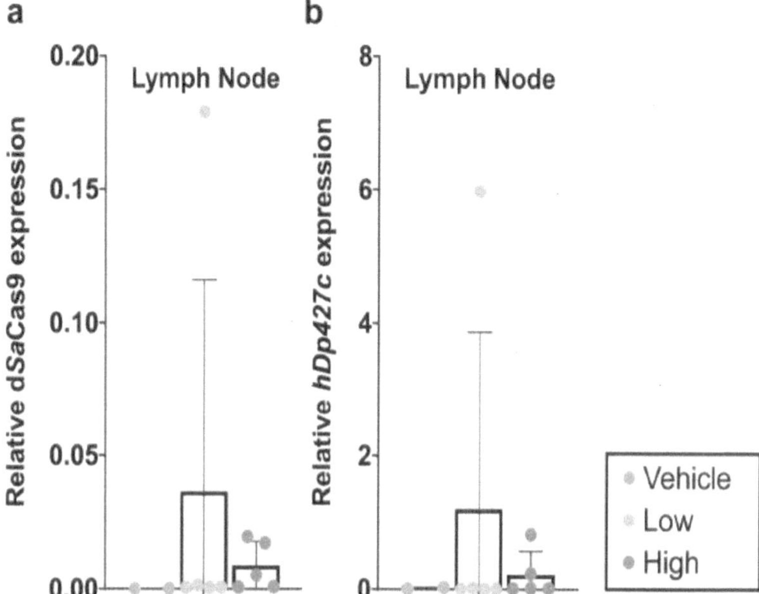

Fig. 3.4.6 **Gene expression in lymph node tissues exhibited high variability. a,** Relative d*Sa*Cas9 expression. **b,** Relative *hDp427c* expression. Mice used to test Andelyn GMP AAV9: Mouse No. Tox1011 & Tox1012 were vehicle-injected control. Mouse No. Tox2011 to Tox2015 were treated with 1e14 vg/kg CRD-TMH-001 (low). Mouse No. Tox3011 to Tox3015 were treated with 2e14 vg/kg CRD-TMH-001 (high). Samples were collected 4 weeks post injection. qPCR standard curves: *hDp427c* (standard curve 3), *mHprt1* (standard curve 3), and d*Sa*Cas9 cDNA (standard curve 3) (Table 3.6.5). qPCR triplicates were performed. Relative *hDp427c* expression was *hDp427c* : *mHprt1*. Relative d*Sa*Cas9 expression was d*Sa*Cas9 (cDNA) : *mHprt1*. Plots depicted mean with SD.

As a summary of this chapter thus far, all the aforementioned results, coupled with pre-clinical findings from our collaborators, were organized and submitted to the FDA. Subsequently, our IND application obtained a "Safe to Proceed" letter from FDA (IND 28497), and the n-of-1 clinical trial, sponsored by Cure Rare Disease, received approval from the institutional review board (IRB) at UMass Medical School. With the written informed consent from Patient1, our clinician collaborators at UMass conducted the clinical trial. (ClinicalTrials.gov: NCT05514249).

3.5 The unexpected death in the clinical trial and post-mortem studies

[This section included a significant amount of work done by our clinician collaborators in order to present a comprehensive overview of this case. Kaiyue Ma did not write all of the text. Refer to Lek *et al.*, 2023 (Author's Note).]

Patient1 (in his 20s) received 1e14 vg/kg of intravenous AAV9 CRD-TMH-001 (IND 28497) at UMass Chan Medical School. At that time, Patient1 had severe muscle weakness with a low lean muscle mass of 45%, a restrictive pulmonary defect, and mild left ventricular (LV) systolic dysfunction. He had been on long term steroid treatment for over two decades. Baseline immunologic screening showed non-detectable AAV9 total antibody and negative ELISPOT responses to AAV9 and the d*Sa*Cas9 fusion protein (1161 aa, including the N-term SV40 NLS, d*Sa*Cas9, nucleoplasmin NLS, VP64, C-term SV40 NLS, and the linkers).

Prophylactic immune suppression therapy was started 13 days prior to dosing. Safety parameters under study included blood counts, serum chemistries, brain natriuretic peptide BNP, and troponin I. Treatment emergent adverse events began 1 day after vector delivery with premature ventricular contractions (PVCs), followed by a downward trend in platelets (2 days post), and increasing BNP (3 days post). Asymptomatic hypercarbia with respiratory acidosis was noted on safety monitoring labs 3-4 days post dose. This resolved with optimizing BiPAP pressures from 10/4 to 12/5.

Five days post dose, Patient1 developed worsening cardiac function presumed to be myopericarditis given elevation in troponin and pericardial effusion with tamponade physiology. Patient1 developed sudden acute respiratory distress 6 days post dose, with CXR findings of acute respiratory distress syndrome (ARDS) and worsening cardiac function. Patient1 progressed to cardiopulmonary arrest and was emergently placed on extracorporeal membrane oxygenation (ECMO). Despite support with ECMO, Patient1 passed away 8 days post-treatment due to multiorgan failure and severe neurological injury.

Laboratory studies from the post-vector period indicated high IL6 (2800 pg/mL) and a mixed picture of complement components with elevated C5b-9. Multiplex cytokine bead-based assays revealed elevations of IL-8 in the serum and high levels of IL-6 and MCP-1 in the pericardial fluid. Mitigating therapies attempted during this time included increased steroids, eculizumab (anti-C5), tocilizumab (anti-IL6-R), and anakinra (IL1-R blocker).

A consent for limited autopsy allowed for gross and microscopic examinations of the heart, lungs, brain, triceps, and liver. The post-mortem examination confirmed markedly decreased muscle mass in the heart and skeletal muscle. Examination of the heart demonstrated severe cardiomyopathy, characterized by significant gross and histologic fibrofatty replacement of biventricular myocardium, consistent with what has been described in dystrophin-deficient cardiomyopathy [376], and without overt features of active inflammation/myocarditis, thrombotic microangiopathy, or complement deposition (confirmed by immunohistochemistry).

The lungs were heavy and edematous (600 gm combined weight, compared with 475 gm expected); the histology showed diffuse alveolar damage, characterized by hyaline membrane formation along with interstitial and intra-alveolar edema.

The findings were in keeping with the clinical impression of ARDS. There was no evidence of thrombotic microangiopathy or significant inflammation. Gross and microscopic examinations of the brain demonstrated infarctions in a "watershed" distribution in the cerebral cortex and cerebellum, and widespread neuronal injury likely reflecting poor perfusion in the pre-terminal stage.

Analyses of AAV vector DNA distribution were performed using qPCR. Vector genomes were detected in lung tissue at a level of 119 vg/diploid genome. Likewise, vector genomes were detected in the myocardium, with 34 vg/diploid genome in the left ventricle sample and 48 vg/diploid genome in the right ventricle sample. Vector genome abundance in liver indicated 680 vg/diploid genome.

The most surprising observation is the substantial distribution of AAV9 in the lung tissue, which was not seen in our pre-clinical mouse study (Fig. 3.4.5f, < ~3 vg/diploid genome for both doses: 1e14 vg/kg & 2e14 vg/kg), in other previous mouse studies [377-379], in dogs [380], or in crab-eating macaques [381]. One intravenous AAV9 study in crab-eating macaques did demonstrate elevated lung biodistribution at one time point [382]; however, the observed level (8e13 vg/kg self-complementary AAV9, 6 months post injection, ~ 20 vg/diploid genome) was still not as high as what we have observed.

Furthermore, a high level of lung biodistribution was also not observed in two other patients in a previous AAV9 clinical trial for Spinal Muscular Atrophy [383] (~ 1 vg/diploid genome for a dose of 1.1e14 vg/kg). We speculated that the biodistribution difference between Patient1 and the other two patients might be due to the short duration post-injection in Patient1 (1 week vs. more than 6 weeks post injection).

Nonetheless, the extent to which this observation of high AAV9 distribution in lung can be generalized remains uncertain. Is it a common trait among all DMD patients, or is it specific to the case of Patient1? It is plausible that the extensive loss of myofibers in Patient1 may have altered the expected vector biodistribution. Above all, the paramount question is whether this had any relevance to the adverse events. More studies are needed to address these questions.

d*Sa*Cas9 transcript expression was assessed using qPCR and revealed no detectable levels in the tissues analyzed except for liver (Fig. 3.5.1a,c). This pattern was also observed for d*Sa*Cas9 protein, as only a faint band was detectable in the liver by western blot. Expression levels of guide-RNA showed similar tissue trends (Fig. 3.5.1b,c). The transgene expression being present in the liver while absent in the heart and skeletal muscle tissues, constituted an unforeseen outcome that defied expectations established by our pre-clinical studies (Fig. 3.4.2 a,c,f,g, Fig. 3.4.5c,h, and Fig. 3.5.1d,e). We speculated that this inconsistency may be partly linked to the difference in time points (1 week *vs.* 4 weeks or later post injection) and the difference in the performance of the hU6 promoter (in human *vs.* in mouse [384,385], Fig. 3.5.1e). However, further studies are required to establish a clearer understanding of this observation. The absence of the transgene in skeletal and cardiac tissues did not warrant measurement of *Dp427c* up-regulation at this timepoint post-mortem (and this measurement is challenging to conduct due to the lack of a suitable control sample).

No AAV9 capsid or Cas9 transgene specific T-cell responses were detected by interferon gamma ELISPOT in Patient1's peripheral blood mononuclear cells (PBMCs) at days 4 or 7 post-dosing.

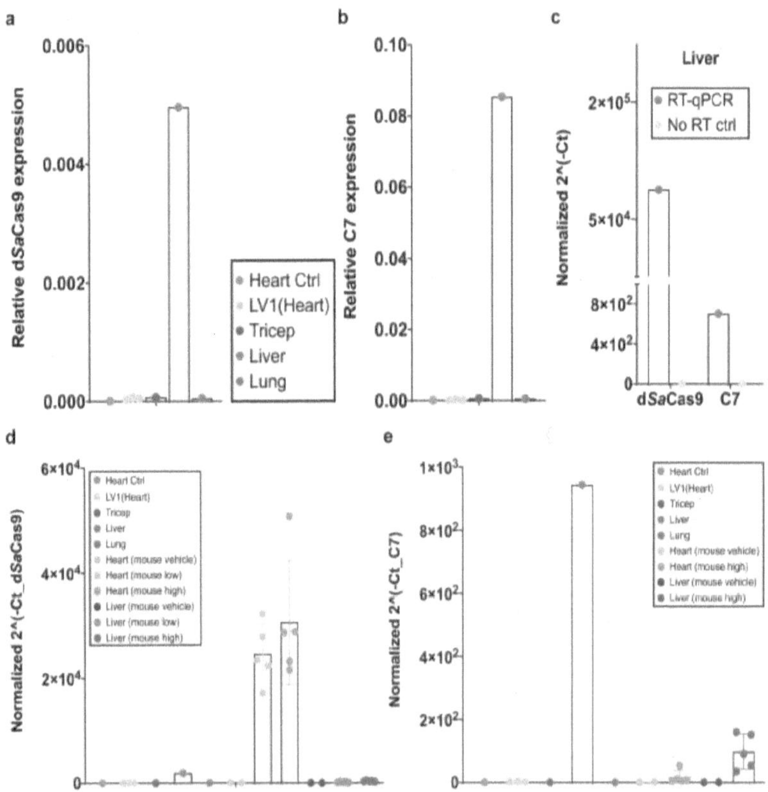

Fig. 3.5.1 Transgene expression in the autopsy samples. a,b, Transgene expression was only detected in liver (**a**, d*Sa*Cas9; **b**, C7 gRNA). qPCR standard curves: *hHPRT1* (standard curve 1) and d*Sa*Cas9 cDNA (standard curve 4) (Table 3.6.5). Relative d*Sa*Cas9 expression was d*Sa*Cas9 (cDNA) : *hHPRT1*. Relative C7 expression was 2^(Ct_*hHPRT1*-Ct_C7). A C7 (primer pair version 2) standard curve could not be generated due to the low expression signal observed in the mouse sample used for creating the standard curves. Heart ctrl: TaKaRa Human Heart Total RNA (TaKaRa, 636532). LV1: heart left ventricular sample1 (this sample piece was sampled at 3 different locations). **c**, RT-qPCR reactions, that induded No-RT (reverse transcriptase) controls, were conducted, confirming that the detected liver signals indeed originated from RNA rather than viral DNA. 2^(-Ct) values were normalized to the No-RT control. **d,e**, A rough comparison of Ct values of d*Sa*Cas9 (**d**) and C7 (**e**) between the autopsy samples and the mouse

samples. [Mouse No. Tox1011 & Tox1012 were vehicle-injected control. Mouse No. Tox2011 to Tox2015 were treated with 1e14 vg/kg CRD-TMH-001 (low). Mouse No. Tox3011 to Tox3015 were treated with 2e14 vg/kg CRD-TMH-001 (high). Samples were collected 4 weeks post injection.] 2^(-Ct) values were normalized to the TaKaRa Heart control (background noise). **c-e**, 20 ng RNA per reaction was used for d*Sa*Cas9 RT-qPCR and 200 ng RNA per reaction for C7. **a-e**, qPCR triplicates were performed. Plots depicted mean with SD (if applicable).

Per our clinic-pathologic findings, we hypothesize Patient1 developed a cytokine-mediated capillary leak syndrome, manifested by pericardial effusion on day 5 and rapidly developing ARDS on day 6. The latter resulted in acute worsening of pulmonary compliance with respiratory failure, hypoxemia, and an associated acute worsening of right ventricle heart failure. Unlike other DMD patients in rAAV trials, this patient did not exhibit evidence of TMA or of adaptive humoral or cell-mediated immune responses to AAV capsid or transgene products.

Another recent fatal case was described in a trial involving a non-ambulatory 16-year-old DMD patient, who passed six days after receiving gene therapy [386]. The patient was part of Pfizer's gene therapy trial (NCT03362502) and received fordadistrogene movaparvovec at 2e14 vg/kg. His death is believed to be linked to an innate immune response against the capsid in the myocardium, which led to cardiogenic shock and heart failure. In our case, we suspected myocarditis clinically because of an acute rise in serum troponins and pericardial effusion. However, the direct histopathological examination of the myocardial tissue post-mortem gave definitive evidence of the absence of innate immune cell infiltration typically seen in myocarditis.

Patient1's late stage of DMD progression at dosing may have limited his physiologic reserves to tolerate the cardiopulmonary stress associated with acute toxicity resulting from rAAV gene therapy, but this was not possible to fully demonstrate.

Capillary leak syndromes have been well-described following cytokine release in other gene and cell therapies, including systemic rAd and CAR-T cell therapies [387-389], but not typically after higher doses of AAV for rare genetic diseases. To our knowledge, this is the first reported case of severe ARDS in AAV gene therapy in DMD. It is possible that this is unique to the specific product; however, since the toxicity occurred prior to detectable levels of transgene expression and since the protein composition of the vector preparations was equivalent to other high-dose AAV9 vectors, it is more likely that this was host-specific rather than vector-specific.

Further research is necessary to investigate host characteristics that render individuals susceptible to severe innate immune reactions to AAV, enhancing the safety of AAV-mediated gene therapy at high doses, particularly for patients with more advanced disease symptoms.

3.6 Materials and Methods for the development of the CRISPRa gene therapy

Institutional approval:

All animal work was performed under the guidelines of Yale University Institutional Animal Care and Use Committee with approved protocols (20270). The Investigational New Drug Application (IND) for CRD-TMH-001 received a "Safe to Proceed" letter issued by the FDA (IND 28497). Patient1 provided written informed consent for the clinical trial study which was sponsored by Cure Rare Disease and performed in accordance with protocols approved by the institutional review board at University of Massachusetts Chan Medical School (ClinicalTrials.gov: NCT05514249).

Mice:

hDMD (Tg(DMD)72Thoen/J, 018900) and mdxD2 (D1.B10-Dmdmdx/J, 013141) mice were initially acquired from The Jackson Laboratory. They were then subjected to crossbreeding to yield the required hDMD/mdxD2 (male) mice for the experiments. The mice were genotyped with corresponding primers.

Mouse No.	Treatment	Sacrifice	Note
20-05	Non-injected	N/A	Female, hDMD/mdxD2
8339	Non-injected	"4 weeks post injection"	
8341			
3001	C (M1): 2.8e13 vg/kg	4 weeks post injection	7e12 vg/kg (Viralgen re-titered)
3002			
3003			
3004			
3005	C (M1): 2.8e14 vg/kg	4 weeks post injection	7e13 vg/kg (Viralgen re-titered)
3006			
3007			
3008			
8365	Non-injected	"8 weeks post injection"	
8377			
3009	C (M1): 2.8e14 vg/kg	8 weeks post injection	
3010			
3011			
3012			
20-38	Non-injected	"8 weeks post injection"	
20-39			
20-42	A (M1): 2.1e14 vg/kg	8 weeks post injection	
20-43	B (M1): 2.1e14 vg/kg		
20-46	A (M1): 1.3e14 vg/kg	8 weeks post injection	
20-47	B (M1): 2.6e14 vg/kg		
20-50	A (M1): 6.1e13 vg/kg	8 weeks post injection	
20-51	B (M1): 3.1e14 vg/kg		
20-81	D (M1): 1e14 vg/kg	4 weeks post injection	
20-82			
20-83			
20-84	Non-injected	"4 weeks post injection"	
20-85			
20-86			
20-106	D (M1): 1e14 vg/kg	12 weeks post injection	
20-107			
20-108			

21-12	Non-injected	"4 weeks post injection"	
21-13			
21-14	D (M2): 2e14 vg/kg	4 weeks post injection	
21-15			
21-16			
21-17			
21-18	DC8 (M2): 1.8e14 vg/kg	4 weeks post injection	
21-19			
21-20			
21-21			
21-22	Non-injected	"4 weeks post injection"	
21-23			
21-24	C (M1): 2.8e14 vg/kg*	4 weeks post injection	*Stored at -80 °C for ~1 year
21-25			
21-26	C (M2): 2e14 vg/kg	4 weeks post injection	4.6e14 vg/kg (Viralgen re-titered)
21-27			
21-28			
21-29			
21-60	Non-injected	"4 weeks post injection"	
21-61			
21-62	C (M1): 2.8e14 vg/kg*	8 weeks post injection	*Stored at -80 °C for ~1 year
21-63	C (M2): 2e14 vg/kg	8 weeks post injection	
21-64			
21-65			
21-66			
21-101	Non-injected	"6 months post injection"	Kept at CRL
21-102			
21-103	C (M2): 2e14 vg/kg	6 months post injection	
21-104			
21-105	Non-injected	"6 months post injection"	Kept at Yale
21-106			
21-108	C (M2): 2e14 vg/kg	6 months post injection	
21-109			
21-110			
21-111			
21-112			
1021	Vehicle injected controls	4 weeks post injection	
1022			
1023			
1024			
1025			
2021	C (M3): 2e13 vg/kg	4 weeks post injection	
2022			
2023			
2024			
2025			
3021	C (M3): 4e13 vg/kg	4 weeks post injection	
3022			
3023			
3024			
3025			

21-212	Non-injected	"4 weeks post injection"	
21-213			
21-214	C (M3): 2.2e14 vg/kg	4 weeks post injection	
21-215			
21-216			
21-217			
2201	Non-injected	"4 weeks post injection"	
2202			
2203	C (M4): 2.5e14 vg/kg	4 weeks post injection	
2204			
2205			
2206			
22-17	L (M2): 1.4e13 vg/kg	4 weeks post injection	B6 WT mice Sex: males
22-18			
22-19			
Tox1011	Vehicle injected controls	4 weeks post injection	
Tox1012			
Tox2011	C (M4): 1e14 vg/kg	4 weeks post injection	The same batch of GMP AAV9 that was utilized in the clinical trial
Tox2012			
Tox2013			
Tox2014			
Tox2015			
Tox3011	C (M4): 2e14 vg/kg	4 weeks post injection	
Tox3012			
Tox3013			
Tox3014			
Tox3015			

Table 3.6.0 "Volunteered heroes": Mice sacrificed for the development of CRD-TMH-001 treatment. For each set of experiments, non-injected mice (if applicable) were sacrificed at the same time as the injected mice. If not otherwise labeled, the mice are male hDMD/mdxD2 mice. A: CMV-dSaCas9-VP64. B: U6-C7-U6-C8-MS2stemloop-EF1α-MCP(N55K)-p65-HSF1. C: CRD-TMH-001. D: CK8e-dual-VP64-C7. DC8: CK8e-dual-VP64-C8. L: AAV serotype library. M1: Manufacturer1, Nationwide Children's Hospital. M2: Manufacturer2, UMass Medical School. M3: Manufacturer3, Viralgen. M4: Manufacturer4, Andelyn. CRL: Charles River Laboratories. The doses were calculated according to the titers reported by the manufacturers.

Cell culture:

HEK293T cells (CRL-3216) were obtained from ATCC. Patient1 fibroblasts were cultured from skin biopsy. The Patient1 iPSC-derived myoblast (iSMS) cell line was established by Dr. Charles P. Emerson's team at UMass Chan Medical School. HEK293T growth medium was made by mixing Dulbecco's Modified Eagle Medium (DMEM) (Gibco, 11966-025), Fetal bovine serum (FBS) (Atlanta Biologicals, S11150; 10% v/v), and Antibiotic-Antimycotic (Gibco, 15240- 062; 1×). Fibroblast growth medium was made by mixing DMEM, FBS (20% v/v), Antibiotic-Antimycotic (1×), and Sodium pyruvate (Gibco, 11360070, 1nM). MB135 growth medium were made by mixing Ham's F10 Nutrient Mix (Gibco, 11550043), FBS (20% v/v), Antibiotic-Antimycotic (1×), FGF (Gibco, PHG0026, 10 ng/mL) and dexamethasone (Sigma, D4902, 10 mM). Other myoblasts were cultured in skeletal muscle growth media (PromoCell, C-23060) supplemented with FBS (20% v/v) and Antibiotic-Antimycotic (1×). To induce myotube formation, myoblasts were switched to skeletal muscle differentiation media (PromoCell, C-23061) supplemented with Antibiotic-Antimycotic (1×).

Plasmid construction:

DNA fragments employed in plasmid construction were obtained through PCR amplification or digestion from existing plasmids (or DNA fragments) using appropriate restriction enzymes. PCR reactions were conducted using either Phusion High-Fidelity DNA Polymerase (NEB, M0530) or Q5 High-Fidelity DNA Polymerase (NEB, M0491SVIAL), following the manufacturer's guidelines. Restriction enzymes were sourced from New England Biolabs (NEB). The assembly of final plasmids using the obtained DNA fragments involved either ligation or Gibson assembly. Ligation reactions utilized T4 ligase (NEB, M0202S), while Gibson assembly reactions employed NEBuilder HiFi DNA Assembly (NEB, E2621S). Tables below present the inventory of generated and/or employed plasmids, as well as the compilation of gRNA sequences utilized in this project.

Backbone	Guide	Note
CMV-d*Sa*Cas9-VPR	C4, C5, C6, P4, P5, P6, BB	The backbone was from: Addgene, 99688
		The U6 cassette was cloned from: Addgene, 99690
CMV-d*Sa*Cas9-VPR-EF1α-BSD	C4, C6, C7, C8, BB	EF1α was from: Addgene, 52963
		BSD was from Addgene, 52962
MHCK7-d*Sa*Cas9-VPR	C4, C6, BB	MHCK7 was cloned from: Addgene, 65042
MHCK7-d*Sa*Cas9-VPR-EF1α-BSD	C4, C6, C7, C8, BB	
EF1α-d*Sa*Cas9-VP64	BB	Obtained from Dr. Sidi Chen's group
CMV-d*Sa*Cas9-VP64	C7, C8, BB	The backbone was from: Addgene, 99680
		The U6 cassette was cloned from: Addgene, 99690
CK8e-d*Sa*Cas9-VP64	C7 (CRD-TMH-001), C8, BB	CK8e was obtained from Dr. Stephen Hauschka's group
		Engineered from: Addgene, 99680
MHCK7-d*Sa*Cas9-VP64	C7, C8, BB	
MS2stemloop-EF1α-MCP(N55K)-p65-HSF1	C6, C7, C8, "C7&C8"	The backbone was obtained from Dr. Sidi Chen's group
MS2stemloop-CK8e-MCP(N55K)-p65-HSF1	C7	
CK8e-eGFP		Engineered from: Addgene, 49055
CMV-VP64-d*Sa*Cas9-VP64	C7, C8	The backbone was from: Addgene, 135338
CK8e-VP64-d*Sa*Cas9-VP64	C7, C8	3×FLAG-tag coding sequence was removed

Table 3.6.1 Plasmids generated and/or used in the development of the CRISPRa gene therapy. Addgene plasmid 99680, 99688, and 99690 were gifts from George Church. Addgene plasmids 52962 and 52963 were gifts from Feng Zhang. MHCK7 is a muscle-specific promoter [390], which was cloned from Addgene plasmid 65042, a gift from Nenad Bursac. "C7&C8": U6-C7 cassette and U6-C8 cassette were cloned into the same plasmid. Addgene plasmid 49055 was a gift from Fred Gage. Addgene plasmid 135338 was a gift from Ronald Cohn. BB: the backbone plasmid without the U6 cassette.

Name	Sequence	Note
C4*	GCTTTGCATCTGTACAGAAGA	gRNA for *Dp427c* up-regulation
C5	TTCTGTACAGATGCAAAGCCT	gRNA for *Dp427c* up-regulation
C6*	TCGACTGACGTATCAGATAGT	gRNA for *Dp427c* up-regulation
C7*	ATCATGCGAAAGGGGAGCTGT	gRNA for *Dp427c* up-regulation
C8*	GGCATGCCCACCTAACCTAAC	gRNA for *Dp427c* up-regulation
P4*	CACCTCACTATTCACGGCAAC	gRNA for *Dp427p* up-regulation
P5*	AAGAAACCATTGCTGTGAGAG	gRNA for *Dp427p* up-regulation
P6*	AACTGTGTCGTCTGCTTTATA	gRNA for *Dp427p* up-regulation

Table 3.6.2 Guide RNAs designed for dystrophin up-regulation. *Patented (PCT/US2020/055089).

Transfection and nucleofection:

Cells were transfected at 70-90% confluency using Lipofectamine 3000 (Thermo Fisher Scientific, L3000-008) according to manufacturer's instructions. Briefly, Lipofectamine 3000 reagent was mixed with half of the Opti-MEM (Gibco, 31985-070) and set aside. In a separate tube the other half of the Opti-MEM was added along with the plasmid DNA and the P300 reagent and pipetted up and down to mix. The

Lipofectamine300/Opti-MEM mix was added to this tube and pipetted to mix. The sample was incubated for 10 minutes (mins) at room temperature (RT) prior and then subsequently added dropwise to the well. The following day (24 hours) the media was replaced with fresh media. An example reaction composition for a well of a 12-well plate is as follows: Plasmid, 2.5 μg; Lipofectamine 3000, 4 μL; Opti-MEM (Gibco, 31985-070), 125 μL; P3000, 5 μL. For nucleofection, plasmids were prepared in SE Cell Line Nucleofector Solution (Lonza, PBC1-00675) and delivered into cells with a Lonza 4D-Nucleofector according to manufacturer's instructions. The program used for HEK293T was EN-138; the program used for fibroblasts was CA-137; The program used for myoblasts was EN-150. An example composition for a well of a 16-well Nucleocuvette Strip is as follows: cells, 100 k; supplemented SE Solution, 30 μL; plasmid, 1-2 μg.

RNA extraction from cells:

RNA extractions were done using the NucleoSpin RNA extraction kit (Takara Bio, 740955.250) according to manufacturer's instructions. To ensure thorough removal of residual DNA in the RNA samples, an additional DNase treatment step was incorporated using the ezDNase kit (Invitrogen, 11766051) following the manufacturer's instructions.

RNA extraction from tissues:

Tissues were added to 1 mL of TRIzol reagent (Life Technologies, 15596018) and homogenized until completely dissolved using a tissue homogenizer (Omni International, 10046-846). Once homogenized they were incubated at room temperature (RT) for 5 mins to permit further dissociation. 200 μL of 1-Bromo-3-chloropropane (VWR, 10841-634) was added and samples were vortexed vigorously then incubated at RT for 2-3 mins. Samples were centrifuged at 12,000 × g 4 °C for 15 mins to separate the RNA, DNA and protein phases. The aqueous RNA phase was carefully removed into a new 1.5 mL microcentrifuge tube and 500 μL of isopropanol (Sigma Aldrich, I9516) was added to precipitate the RNA. Samples were inverted to ensure thorough mixing and then incubated at RT for 10 mins. Following this, they were centrifuged at 12,000 × g for 15 mins at 4 °C. The supernatant was discarded, and the pellet was washed twice with 75% ethanol. After each wash, the sample was centrifuged at 10,000 × g for 10 mins at 4 °C. The supernatant was removed, and the pellet was air dried for 10 mins at RT. Subsequently, the RNA pellet was reconstituted in nuclease-free water, adjusted based on pellet size (50-800 μL). The RNA samples underwent treatment with the ezDNase kit (Invitrogen, 11766051) prior to their utilization in subsequent steps.

DNA extraction:

DNA extraction from both cells and tissues was accomplished using the Invitrogen PureLink Genomic DNA Mini Kit (Thermo Fisher Scientific, K182001), following the appropriate protocols outlined in the manual. For tissue samples, an appropriate-sized piece was excised using a sterile disposable scalpel (VWR, 500348), and then minced to augment the surface area to achieve optimal digestion.

RT-PCR, RT-qPCR and qPCR:

RT-PCR, RT-qPCR, and qPCR were performed following manufacturers' manuals. RNA was reverse transcribed to cDNA using PrimeScript RT Reagent Kit (Takara Bio, RR037A). Phusion High-Fidelity DNA Polymerase (NEB, M0530) or Q5 High-Fidelity DNA Polymerase (NEB, M0491SVIAL) was used for PCR reactions. SsoAdvanced Universal SYBR Green Supermix (Bio-Rad, 1725271) or iTaq Universal SYBR Green One-Step Kit (Bio-Rad, 1725151), Hard-Shell 96-Well PCR Plates (Bio-Rad, HSP9601), Plate Sealing Film (Bio-Rad, MSB1001) and Bio-Rad C1000 Touch Thermal Cycler were used for RT-qPCR/qPCR experiments. In general, the RT-qPCR used 20 ng (d*Sa*Cas9) or 200 ng (others) RNA (or equivalent amount of cDNA) as input per 20 μL reaction. For qPCR reactions involving genomic DNA as input, a general guideline was to use approximately 40 ng per 20 μL reaction. Primers and qPCR conditions are detailed in the tables provided below.

Name	Note	Sequence	Purpose
Dp427c_F	1	aggagaaagatgctgttttgca	RT-(q)PCR for *Dp427c* (149 bp) and human-specific *Dp427c* (366 bp
Dp427p_F		cagcaaaaagctttcctatgaagg	RT-(q)PCR for *Dp427p* (*p1*: 127 bp; *p2*:211 bp)
Dp427R		aaattgtgcatttacccatttgtg	RT-(q)PCR for *Dp427c* (149 bp)
			RT-(q)PCR for *Dp427m* (177 bp)
			RT-(q)PCR for *Dp427p* (*p1*: 127 bp; *p2*:211 bp); not recommended
GAPDHF		gaaggtgaaggtcggagtca	RT-(q)PCR for *GAPDH* (117 bp)
GAPDHR		ttgaggtcaatgaaggggtc	RT-(q)PCR for *GAPDH* (117 bp)
mDp427cF	1	aggagaaagatgctgttttgcg	RT-(q)PCR for mouse (-specific) *Dp427c* (149 bp/305 bp)
mDp427cR		aaattgtgcatttatccatttgtg	RT-(q)PCR for mouse *Dp427c* (149 bp, based on XM_006527768.4)
dSaCas9F		ctacgaggccagagtgaagg	PCR/ RT-(q)PCR for *Sa*Cas9 (192 bp)
dSaCas9R		tcggccacgtatttctcttc	PCR/ RT-(q)PCR for *Sa*Cas9 (192 bp)
p65-F		cgaggggactctgagtgaag	PCR/ RT-(q)PCR for p65 (198 bp, as in Addgene 119074)
p65-R		gggtactccatcagcattgg	PCR/ RT-(q)PCR for p65 (198 bp, as in Addgene 119074)
hDp427m-F	1	tctcattgtttttaagccta	RT-(q)PCR for *Dp427m* (177 bp)
			RT-(q)PCR for human-specific *Dp427m* (394 bp)
hDp427-R	1	catctacgatgtcagtacttcca	RT-(q)PCR for human-specific *Dp427m* (394 bp) and *Dp427c* (366 b
mDp427m-F	1	tctcatcgtacctaagcctc	RT-(q)PCR for mouse-specific *Dp427m* (336 bp)
mDp427-R	1	cagtgccttgttgacattgttcag	RT-(q)PCR for mouse-specific *Dp427m* (336 bp)
			RT-(q)PCR for mouse-specific *Dp427c* (305 bp, XM_006527768.4)
mHprt1-F		caaactttgctttccctggt	RT-(q)PCR for mouse *Hprt1* (101 bp)
mHprt1-R		tctggcctgtatccaacacttc	RT-(q)PCR for mouse *Hprt1* (101 bp)
hDMDgt-F	2	cttgtggggacaagaaatcg	Genotyping for hDMD mice (457 bp)
hDMDgt-R	2	caggcttcccaatttttcct	Genotyping for hDMD mice (457 bp)

p9427	3	aactcatcaaatatgcgtgttagtg	Genotyping for mdx mice (105 bp)
p259E	3	gtcactcagatagttgaagccatttaa	Genotyping for mdx mice (with mdx mutation) (105 bp)
p260E	3	gtcactcagatagttgaagccatttag	Genotyping for mdx mice (without mdx mutation) (105 bp)
Ltbp4-F	4	aaccgctacccaaaccttca	Genotyping for the D2 background (D2: 353 bp/non-D2: 389 bp)
Ltbp4-R	4	aggctttctgcctactcgtc	Genotyping for the D2 background (D2: 353 bp/non-D2: 389 bp)
Abcc-F	5	tgtatctccaggctcgagtg	Genotyping for the D2 background (192 bp)
Abcc-R	5	ggtaccaagtgacacgacag	Genotyping for the D2 background (192 bp)
C7RTPCRv1F		accgatcatgcgaaaggggagctgt	Version1, not recommended: RT-(q)PCR for C7 gRNA (121 bp)
C7RTPCRv1R		ggcgtctcagaccaaaaaaatctcgccaacaagttgacgag	Version1, not recommended: RT-(q)PCR for C7 gRNA (121 bp)
C7RTPCRv2F		gatcatgcgaaaggggagc	Version2: RT-(q)PCR for C7 gRNA (98 bp)
C7RTPCRv2R		tctcgccaacaagttgacg	Version2: RT-(q)PCR for C7 gRNA (98 bp)
WPRE-F		gggacgtccttctgctacg	qPCR for constructs carrying WPRE (122 bp)
WPRE-R		gagatccgactcgtctgagg	qPCR for constructs carrying WPRE (122 bp)
CK8e-F		cccatgtaaggaggcaagg	qPCR (193 bp); not recommended, mouse native band: 1045 bp
CK8e-R		ctgacttgctcactggttcc	qPCR (193 bp); not recommended, mouse native band: 1045 bp
Dp427ex23F		aagcgccctctgaaattagc	RT-(q)PCR for *Dp427* (*Dp427c*, *Dp427m*, & *Dp427p*; 171 bp)
Dp427ex24R		cagccatccatttcttcagg	RT-(q)PCR for *Dp427* (*Dp427c*, *Dp427m*, & *Dp427p*; 171 bp)
KIAA1217-F		tcaagtgggagaggctgtagct	RT-(q)PCR for *KIAA1217* (144 bp)
KIAA1217-R		acacgcttcaggagactgtcca	RT-(q)PCR for *KIAA1217* (144 bp)
SSX2IP-F		gactttgccagacacgttcctg	RT-(q)PCR for *SSX2IP* (135 bp)
SSX2IP-R		aggtcttgatgccacactccat	RT-(q)PCR for *SSX2IP* (135 bp)
UGGT1-F		ggacggcagttactgtatgatgc	RT-(q)PCR for *UGGT1* (162 bp)
UGGT1-R		cttagcagcgttggaagtctgag	RT-(q)PCR for *UGGT1* (162 bp)
hHPRT1-F		cattatgctgaggatttggaaagg	RT-(q)PCR for *hHPRT1* (129 bp)
hHPRT1-R		cttgagcacacagagggctaca	RT-(q)PCR for *hHPRT1* (129 bp)

Table 3.6.3 Primers used in the development of the CRISPRa gene therapy. (1), the primers were also used in a previous publication [367]. (2), a protocol is available from The Jackson Laboratory (29160). (3), the primers were designed in a previous study [391]. (4), the primers were also used in a previous study [392]. (5), a protocol is available from TREAT-NMD (DMD_M.2.2.005).

Reagent	**Amount**	**Reagent**	**Amount**
cDNA/gDNA	x μL	RNA	x μL
10 μM Forward primer	0.5 μL	10 μM Forward + Reverse primer mix	1 μL
10 μM Reverse primer	0.5 μL	Reverse transcriptase	0.25 μL
Sso Advanced SYBR green mastermix	10 μL	iTaq reaction mix	10 μL
nuclease free water	to 20 μL	nuclease free water	to 20 μL

qPCR			**RT-qPCR**		
Temperature	**Time**	**Cycles**	**Temperature**	**Time**	**Cycles**
95 °C	3 mins	1	50 °C	10 mins	1
95 °C	10 s	39 (plate read)	95 °C	3 mins	1
A/E Temp.	A/E Time		95 °C	10 s	39 (plate read)
			A/E Temp.	A/E Time	

Primers used for qPCRs		
Primer pairs	A/E temperature	A/E time
Dp427c (149 bp)	**55 °C**	**30 s**
Dp427m (177 bp)	55 °C	30 s
	53 °C	30 s
Dp427 (171 bp)	55 °C	30 s
GAPDH (117 bp)	**55 °C**	**30 s**
mHprt1 (101 bp)	**57 °C**	**1 min**
	55 °C	30 s

hHPRT1 (129 bp)	**57 °C**	**1 min**
hDp427m (394 bp)	55 °C	30 s
	53 °C	1 min 10 s
hDp427c (366 bp)	**57 °C**	**1 min**
	55 °C	30 s
mDp427m (336 bp)	55 °C	30 s
mDp427c (305 bp)	55 °C	30 s
dSaCas9 (192 bp)	**57 °C (RNA)**	**1 min (RNA)**
	55 °C (DNA)	**30 s (DNA)**
mdx (105 bp)	**55 °C**	**30 s**
CK8e (193 bp)	55 °C	30 s
C7 version 1 (121 bp)	**57 °C**	**1 min**
	55 °C	30 s
C7 version 2 (98 bp)	**57 °C**	**1 min**
KIAA1217 (144 bp)	55 °C	30 s
SSX2IP (135 bp)	55 °C	30 s
UGGT1 (162 bp)	55 °C	30 s

Table 3.6.4 qPCR/RT-qPCR conditions used in the development of the CRISPRa gene therapy. A/E: annealing/extension. Certain pairs of primers were employed under various conditions while maintaining their specificity in those respective settings. In cases where standard curves were established, they were generated to the specific conditions in use. The **bold** conditions were utilized in the pre-clinical and clinical experiments.

Standard curves:

Standard curves were generated using serially diluted samples containing the template of interest for qPCR reactions, allowing the establishment of a function relating the qPCR Ct value to the abundance of the template. The range of Ct values (x) for the standard curves was carefully chosen to accommodate the Ct values of the actual samples. The values representing the template abundance (y) in the standard curves were either arbitrary (used for gene expression quantification) or well-defined (used for biodistribution analysis). To establish the standard curves for gDNA input (*e.g.*, mdx primers), the samples were measured using a NanoDrop 2000 spectrophotometer. To establish the standard curves for viral copy number (*e.g.*, d*Sa*Cas9 primers), the plasmid template was initially diluted to ~1 ng/μL (NanoDrop) and then quantified using the

Qubit 1X dsDNA High Sensitivity (HS) Assay Kit (Invitrogen, Q33230) to acquire the precise concentration. The viral copy number was calculated using the following equation (The molecular weight was obtained using Sequence Manipulation Suite->Sequence Analysis->DNA Molecular Weight [393]):

$$Viral\_copy\_number = plasmid\_weight * 2 * Avogadro\ constant/plasmid\_molecular\_weight$$

Stand curves	**Functions**	**Standard "1"**
hDp427c standard curve 1	6091358196.49552*EXP(1)^(-0.8274494919*Ct)	50 ng Mouse No. 3012 heart RNA
hDp427c standard curve 2	5789392.44987157*EXP(1)^(-0.7079562612*Ct)	200 ng Mouse No. 20-05 brain RNA
hDp427c standard curve 3	268247.692706032*EXP(1)^(-0.5896758914*Ct)	200 ng Mouse No. 20-05 brain RNA
mHprt1 standard curve 1	3291577.90088362*EXP(1)^(-0.7063224256*Ct)	50 ng Mouse No. 3012 heart RNA
mHprt1 standard curve 2	50512.4625008089*EXP(1)^(-0.6867898493*Ct)	200 ng Mouse No. 20-05 brain RNA
mHprt1 standard curve 3	130328.731856329*EXP(1)^(-0.7235008478*Ct)	200 ng Mouse No. 20-05 brain RNA
hHPRT1 standard curve 1	6720571.73179894*EXP(1)^(-0.6080430546*Ct)	200 ng Human Heart Total RNA
		TaKaRa, 636532
d*Sa*Cas9 (cDNA) standard curve 1	56733.8262282853*EXP(1)^(-0.7292004965*Ct)	50 ng Mouse No. 3012 heart RNA
d*Sa*Cas9 (cDNA) standard curve 2	62.2900776189*EXP(1)^(-0.6593479257*Ct)	1 ng CRD-TMH-001 plasmid
d*Sa*Cas9 (cDNA) standard curve 3	74175.2202958675*EXP(1)^(-0.7343217072*Ct)	200 ng Mouse No. 2203 heart RNA
d*Sa*Cas9 (cDNA) standard curve 4	4006.5765672931*EXP(1)^(-0.6374394874*Ct)	200 ng Mouse No. Tox3011 heart RNA
d*Sa*Cas9 sequence standard curve 1	45458409382.6469*EXP(1)^(-0.6816184646*Ct)	1 viral copy
d*Sa*Cas9 sequence standard curve 2	40360909417.4989*EXP(1)^(-0.6555342164*Ct)	1 viral copy
mdx sequence standard curve 1	(4.0822327995*EXP(1)^(-0.7653000308*Ct))*1e6	1 µg mouse gDNA input
mdx sequence standard curve 2	23898124.7817897*EXP(1)^(-0.7751815354*Ct)	1 µg mouse gDNA input
C7 version1 standard curve 1	160217966278.126*EXP(1)^(-0.4651386002*Ct)	1 copy

Table 3.6.5 Functions derived from standard curves. The equations were generated using the exponential trendline option in Microsoft Excel. Different batches of primers were used for different standard curves.

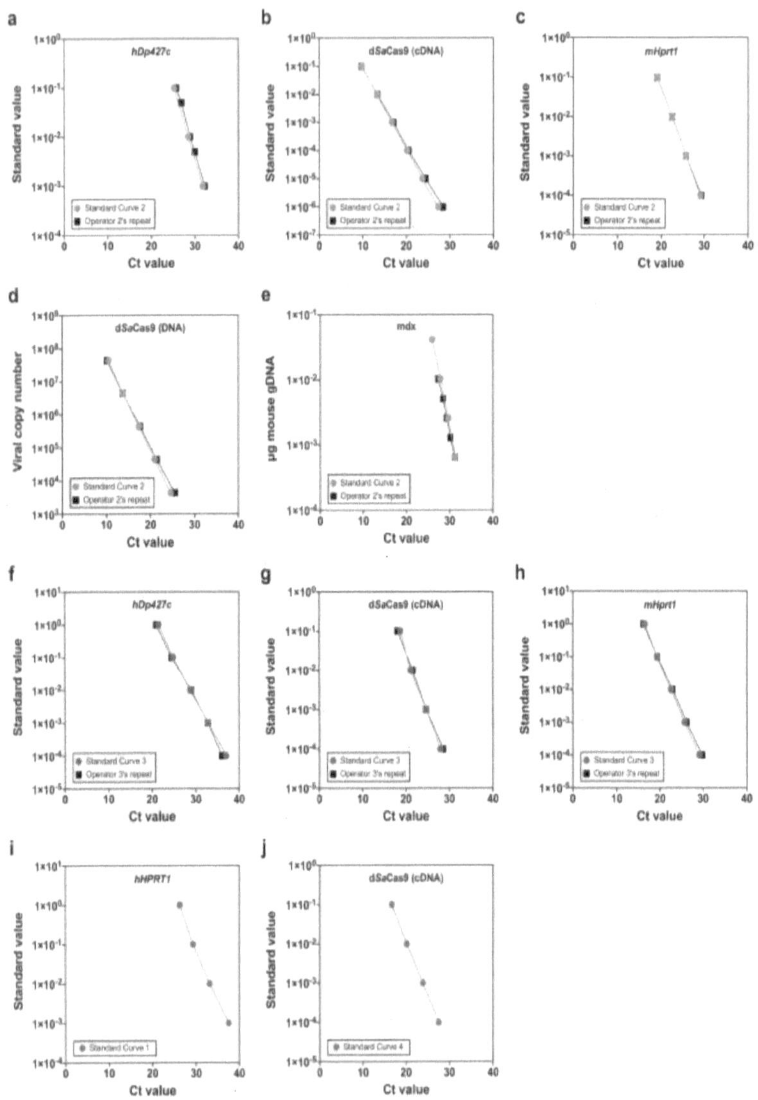

Fig. 3.6.6 Example standard curves. a-h, Error bars depict SD. Operator 2: A. DeSimone. Operator 3: S. Huang.

<u>Examining on-site indels and integration events:</u>

While they are unlikely to occur in the dCas9 context, Sanger sequencing and NGS (Amplicon-EZ) were conducted for PCR products of the C7 region to confirm the absence of indels and on-site integration events.

Primers Used				
Sanger-F	TGTTTGCTCCGAGGTATAGG		250 bp	
Sanger-R	TGCAAAACAGCATCTTTCTCC			
NGS-F1	gcacaaaaggaaactcaccctTAGGCATGCCCACCTAACC			
NGS-R1	cgactcggtgccactttttcTGCAAAACAGCATCTTTCTCC			
NGS-F2	[adaptor+barcode]gcacaaaaggaaactcaccct			
NGS-R2	[adaptor+barcode]cgactcggtgccactttttc			
PCR for Sanger sequencing				
Q5 Rxn	10 μL	1	98 °C	hot start
Q5 Enh	10 μL	2	98 °C	3 mins
10 mM dNTPs	1 μL	3	98 °C	8 s
10 μM F	2.5 μL	4	64 °C	15 s
10 μM R	2.5 μL	5	72 °C	2 mins
gDNA	100 ng	6	Repeat 3-5 for 34 more cycles	
Q5	0.5 μL	7	72 °C	5 mins
Water	To 50 μL	8	4 °C	Forever
PCR purification with NucleoSpin Gel and PCR Clean-Up Kit (Takara, 740609).				
PCR1 for NGS				
Q5 Rxn	10 μL	1	98 °C	hot start
Q5 Enh	10 μL	2	98 °C	3 mins
10 mM dNTPs	1 μL	3	98 °C	8 s
10 μM F	2.5 μL	4	64 °C	15 s
10 μM R	2.5 μL	5	72 °C	5 mins
gDNA	100 ng	6	Repeat 3-5 for 27 more cycles	
Q5	0.5 μL	7	72 °C	5 mins
Water	To 50 μL	8	12 °C	Forever
PCR purification with NucleoSpin Gel and PCR Clean-Up Kit (Takara, 740609).				
PCR2 for NGS				
Q5 Rxn	10 μL	1	98 °C	hot start
Q5 Enh	10 μL	2	98 °C	3 mins
10 mM dNTPs	1 μL	3	98 °C	6 s
10 μM F	2.5 μL	4	67 °C	15 s
10 μM R	2.5 μL	5	72 °C	5 mins
Purified PCR1 product	100 ng	6	Repeat 3-5 for 32 more cycles	
Q5	0.5 μL	7	72 °C	5 mins
Water	To 50 μL	8	12 °C	Forever
Gel purification with NucleoSpin Gel and PCR Clean-Up Kit (Takara, 740609).				

Table 3.6.7 Examine the genomic region flanking the C7 cite. Adaptor: Illumina sequencing adaptors. Scripts are available: https://github.com/leklab/DMD_projects_KM.

3.7 A summary of the established trajectory for n-of-1 gene therapy development

The CRD-TMH-001 clinical trial concluded with a heartbreaking outcome. As scientists and team members deeply engaged in this endeavor, we were shattered and profoundly saddened by the abrupt termination of a once-promising aspiration, cruelly disrupted by the harsh realities of the situation. We have been persistently scrutinizing the entire developmental process and continuously posing the question to ourselves: What could we have done better? This introspection carries on to this day and will continue in the foreseeable future, as we consider it our responsibility to Patient1, other patients, and the entire rare disease community.

Amid the prevailing sense of sorrow, we found solace in the messages from many patient families. They told us that our story had ignited hope, as our project established a new, rapid, and precise development trajectory for individualized gene therapy, all without dependence on large pharmaceutical companies. Learning that our work continues to imbue the community with hope, despite the outcomes, was truly heartening. Indeed, the research of CRD-TMH-001 unfolded rapidly. From muscle biopsy, whole-genome sequencing (WGS), and RNA-seq for Patient1 to the AAV9 dosing clinical trial, the entire journey took approximately four years (Fig. 3.7.1). This was the product of collaborative efforts from an extensive team, uniting scientists, medical doctors from many institutes, contract research organizations, patient foundations, and regulatory teams. By delegating tasks in the drug development process to experts in their respective domains, the rapid development of individualized drugs can be made attainable.

However, on the other hand, we also recognize that there were several aspects during the journey that could have been improved. We aim to outline these aspects here not to dwell on what could have been, but rather to highlight the lessons we have learned and contribute to the ongoing enhancement of the drug development trajectory.

There were two significant setbacks during our journey, both of which could have been managed more efficiently to save time. The first setback was related to the extended evaluation period of the dual-VP64 system, which unexpectedly exhibited low *in vivo* performance (3.3.2). We eventually had to abandon it and revert to the single-VP64 system. Such unforeseeable issues may continue to arise in future gene therapy developments. However, we did gain some valuable insights from this experience: firstly, testing multiple candidate constructs simultaneously could expedite the process, and secondly, caution should be exercised when designing AAV constructs containing repetitive elements. The second setback arose during the manufacturing of the initial batch of GMP (Good Manufacturing Practice) AAV9, which did not yield a sufficient concentration/quantity for the clinical trial. This situation can be prevented in future developments through careful selection of manufacturers and improved communication with them.

Another significant point to highlight is that we were unable to conduct drug safety and efficacy research using a patient-specific mouse strain prior to the clinical trial. Instead, we had to utilize a healthy humanized mouse strain (hDMD/mdxD2) to evaluate the safety and efficacy of the *hDp427c* up-regulation. The primary reason for this was the extended time required to develop the patient-specific mouse strain (Fig. 3.7.1).

However, upon reflection, we recognized that if the process of creating such a mouse strain had commenced earlier, it could have potentially been available for research purposes before the clinical trial.

Time is a luxury that patients with severe rare diseases often cannot afford [394]. Contrary to what one may assume, living with a rare disease is more than just a significant inconvenience in life; it is a ticking time bomb that often correlates with high fatality rates and early deaths [1]. As researchers, we are committed to expediting therapy development while ensuring the validity of results. With an increasing number of clinical trials being initiated, we hold the belief that a faster and more standardized trajectory can be established and adopted by the field for the future development of individualized therapies.

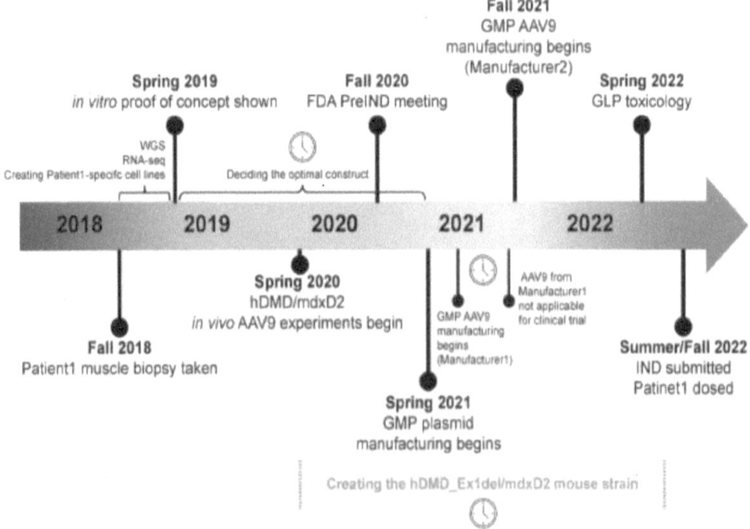

Fig. 3.7.1 The development process of CRD-TMH-001. GMP: Good Manufacturing Practice. GLP: Good Laboratory Practice. Clock icons indicate the stages that could have been further improved.

3.8 Towards safer and more effective and affordable gene therapies

High AAV doses are often associated with severe adverse events [48395396] (3.5). However, in the case of CRD-TMH-001, a high dose was required to effectively achieve *Dp427c* up-regulation (3.4). One strategy to enhance the up-regulation level is to utilize a stronger activator. Although such options were not available during the development of treatment for Patient1, they are now made possible by the recent development of dCasMINI-VPR [300], which can be incorporated into an AAV vector (as demonstrated in one of our designs: 4505 bp between ITRs). By utilizing our CK8e-dCasMINI-VPR construct, we were able to achieve a notably higher level of dystrophin up-regulation in comparison to the d*Sa*Cas9-single-VP64 or the d*Sa*Cas9-dual-VP64 constructs. Currently, we are evaluating its *in vivo* performance. We are also in the process of addressing the question of whether utilizing a stronger activator can enable the use of a smaller dose to achieve equivalent therapeutic effects (Fig. 3.8.1), thereby enhancing the safety of gene therapy.

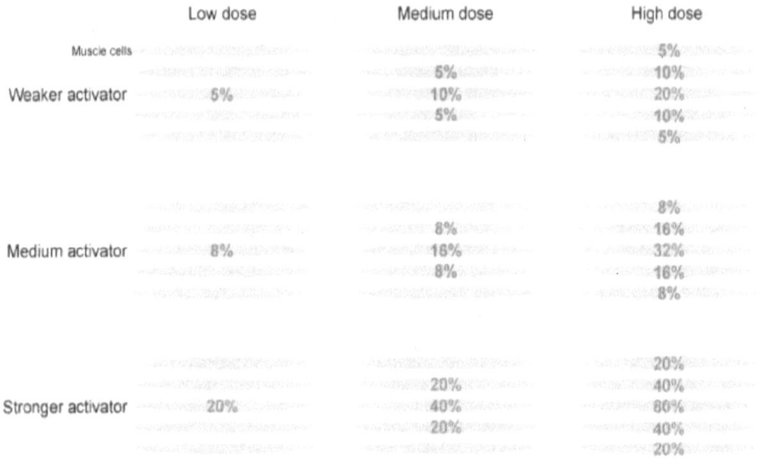

Muscle cells	Low dose	Medium dose	High dose
Weaker activator	5%	5% 10% 5%	5% 10% 20% 10% 5%
Medium activator	8%	8% 16% 8%	8% 16% 32% 16% 8%
Stronger activator	20%	20% 40% 20%	20% 40% 80% 40% 20%

Fig. 3.8.1 Using a stronger activator may or may not result in a reduction of the required AAV dose to achieve therapeutic benefits. For the up-regulation to have a significant physiological impact, a certain proportion of the muscle cells need to attain up-regulation levels above a specific threshold. Consequently, even when employing a relatively stronger activator, it's conceivable that a relatively high dose might still be necessary to achieve therapeutic benefits. The numbers here, which indicate dystrophin up-regulation levels, are merely used as examples.

Another primary reason for the necessity of a high AAV9 dose in muscle diseases is that a significant portion of the viral particles fail to be delivered to the muscle tissues [397]. Therefore, another strategy to reduce the required AAV dose for muscle disease gene therapy is to develop novel engineered AAV serotypes that exhibit higher specificity for muscle tissues. This approach has been recently realized through the creation of MyoAAV and AAVMYO, both of which employed capsid myotropic peptide insertion and demonstrated improved muscle specificity compared to AAV9 [398,399]. We tested four novel serotypes reported in the MyoAAV study, and they indeed demonstrated improved muscle specificity in our experiments (Fig. 3.8.2).

More recently, an updated version of AAVMYO called AAVMYO2 was developed, featuring a shuffled capsid sequence along with myotropic peptide insertion [400]. It has been reported to exhibit even lower liver enrichment compared to AAVMYO. Currently, in our lab, we are using AAVMYO2 for various gene therapy research projects.

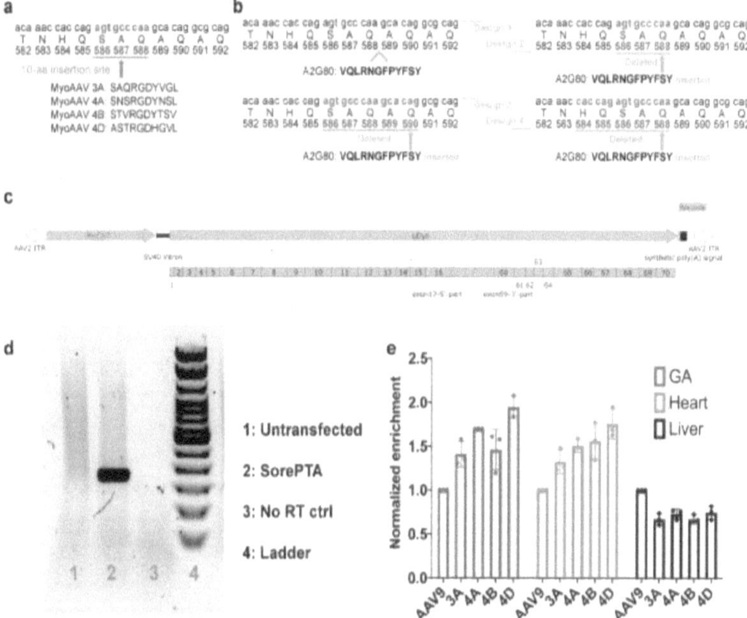

Fig. 3.8.2 Preliminary tests for the MyoAAV serotypes. The MyoAAV viral particles were packaged at University of Massachusetts Medical School. **a**, The MyoAAV serotypes we tested. The sequences were obtained from the publication of the MyoAAV study [398]. To create the MyoAAV Rep-Cap plasmid, three amino acids (586-588) were removed from the Cap sequence on the pAAV2/9 plasmid (obtained from Dr. Jun Xie, UMass), and the MyoAAV 10-aa peptide was inserted at this location (between 585 and 589). **b**, We also attempted four whimsical designs in an effort to insert the α-DG binding peptide A2G80 [401,402] into the same location. All four failed to package. **c**, For the cargo employed in these tests, we generated a micro-dystrophin construct. The micro-dystrophin sequence was obtained from Addgene plasmid 26810, a gift from Jeffrey Chamberlain [403]. The synthetic poly(A) signal was from a previous publication [404]. Barcode sequences were incorporated between the stop codon and the poly(A) signal to differentiate between different serotypes. Since our construct utilized the same MHCK7 promoter and seemingly the same exons as Sarepta's SRP-9001 [322,405,406], we named our construct "SorePTA". udys: micro-dystrophin. **d**, MB135 was transfected with the SorePTA construct using Lipofectamine 3000. RT-PCR was performed using the RNA from the transfected cells. F: atgctttggtgggaagaagt. R: catctacgatgtcagtacttcca. No RT ctrl: SorePTA-transfected MB135 RNA without reverse transcription. **e**, We mixed different AAV serotypes and administered the mixed AAV to 3 mice (Mouse No. 22-17 to 22-19, 4 wks post injection). The enrichment of serotypes was quantified by utilizing Amplicon-EZ NGS on DNA extracted from the gastrocnemius (GA), heart, and liver tissues. The enrichment of a serotype is calculated as the ratio of its

proportion in the tissue DNA to its proportion in the mixed AAV particles, normalized to AAV9 enrichment. Scripts are available: https://github.com/leklab/DMD_projects_KM.

Besides safety and efficacy concerns, another significant issue associated with AAV is the exorbitant cost of manufacturing [407-409]. Despite continuous efforts to improve production efficiency and cost-effectiveness [410-412], the current market price of AAV and AAV-based gene therapy drugs remains beyond the reach of ordinary families. However, diseases do not discriminate between the rich and the poor. A cheaper solution is imperative!

Antibody-oligo conjugates represent an emerging field of research that holds promise in addressing several challenges linked to AAV [413,414]. Given the diverse design possibilities of such conjugates, this non-viral delivery approach may hold the potential to improve muscle delivery, enable redosing, and most importantly, offer a markedly more cost-effective gene therapy strategy.

Two current drugs, Avidity AOC1001 and DYNE-101, both comprised of a monoclonal antibody conjugate to the transferrin receptor (TfR), have been shown to have some success in clinical trials for myotonic dystrophy [415]. However, these antibodies are still constrained by their large size and dependence on mammalian models for production. In contrast, synthetic nanobodies have the potential to overcome these limitations, given their considerably smaller size and the ability to be programmatically designed and readily synthesized using *Escherichia coli* [416,417].

Currently, in the lab, we are investigating the use of an anti-TfR nanobody for delivering oligos to muscle cells and tissues (Fig. 3.8.3). We also have plans to generate additional nanobodies to target other muscle-specific antigens (*e.g.*, CACNG1, CACNG6, and ITGA7) for precise and targeted delivery.

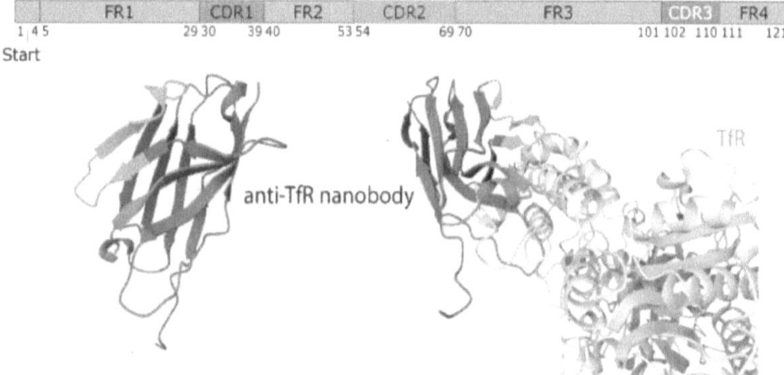

Fig. 3.8.3 An example anti-TfR nanobody. The 3D structures were predicted using Alphafold2 [418].

Chapter 4: Future prospect and novel therapeutic opportunities

Our approach to addressing the challenges presented by rare diseases is in a constant state of evolution. With the continuous advancement of biotechnology, new diagnostic methods are emerging, enabling more accurate and timely identification of the underlying genetic pathology mechanisms. Complementing these efforts are increasingly sophisticated functional assays that provide insights into the molecular-level mechanisms driving these disorders.

Furthermore, our capacity to acquire and translate genetic insights into therapeutic opportunities is expanding. The integration of diverse disciplines, spanning genomics, bioinformatics, molecular biology, and clinical research, is propelling a collaborative effort to untangle the intricacies of rare diseases and foster substantial enhancements in patient outcomes.

4.1 long-read sequencing in diagnostics and discovery of novel genetic mechanisms

4.1.1 The emergence and promises of long-read sequencing

The emergence of long-read sequencing represents a significant breakthrough in biomedical research [419] and has elevated read lengths to a routine 10-kb level [420].

There are two major technical paths to achieve long-read sequencing [421]. One is exemplified by the single molecule real-time (SMRT) sequencing technology from Pacific Biosciences (PacBio) [422], and the other is nanopore sequencing exemplified by the technology from Oxford Nanopore Technologies (ONT) [423,424].

In SMRT, a pair of hairpin sequencing adaptors (SMRTbell) is introduced at the ends of double-stranded DNA (dsDNA) molecules with the desired long lengths. A DNA polymerase, along with a primer targeting the SMRTbell sequence, is added to the DNA library. Subsequently, the prepared library is added into the SMRT Cell within the sequencer. The SMRT cell comprises millions of tiny wells known as zero-mode waveguides (ZMW) [425]. These ZMWs are cavities with diameters in the tens of nanometers, fabricated within a 100-nm thick metal film deposited on a glass substrate [425,426]. Each ZMW accommodates a single molecule of DNA. The polymerase, bound to the DNA, is anchored to the bottom glass surface of the ZMW, immobilizing the polymerase-DNA complex [427]. As the polymerase incorporates fluorophore-labeled nucleotides, the fluorophore emits light. In SMRT, nucleotides contain a fluorescent label on the phosphate chain rather than on the base. Incorporated nucleotides are detected based on the associated fluorophore, which is released and dissipated upon cleavage of the phosphate chain, a natural step in DNA synthesis. Laser light directed through the glass into the ZMW illuminates only its lower 30 nm portion, since the ZMW dimensions are smaller than the wavelength of the light [425]. This allows the selective excitation and identification of the fluorophore-labeled nucleotides that are being held by the polymerase for fractions of a second [428]. SMRT offers two sequencing strategies: Circular Consensus Sequencing (CCS), which generates accurate long reads (HiFi Reads) [429], and Continuous Long Read (CLR) sequencing, which can produce the longest possible reads achievable with SMRT [430].

In the ONT technology, the core element is a nanopore. While most of the specific nanopore proteins used by ONT were not disclosed, it has been reported that the R9 versions utilized the nanopore derived from Curlin sigma S-dependent growth subunit G (CsgG) from *Escherichia coli* [431-433]. In the ONT systems, the protein nanopore is inserted to an electrically resistant membrane, such as a lipid bilayer membrane [423] or a synthetic polymer membrane [434,435]. Future generations of nanopores may be fabricated from synthetic materials, independent from nanopore proteins. For instance, solid-state nanopores are nanometer-sized holes formed in a synthetic membrane, typically made of materials such as SiNx or SiO2 [436,437]. In long-read sequencing, two ionic solution-filled chambers are separated by the nanopore membrane. The dsDNA to be sequenced is mixed with a processive enzyme, capable of processing it into individual single polynucleotide strands. The processive enzyme, derived from a helicase (or polymerase or nuclease), also serves as a motor protein to control the translocation of the DNA strand through the nanopore [438-442]. The DNA-motor protein complex is recruited to the nanopores through the binding of the adapter at the leading end of the DNA to the tethering oligos, which are localized proximal to the nanopore [443]. The two strands of the dsDNA are linked by a hairpin at the far end to the nanopore, enabling the sequencing of the second strand after the first strand has been sequenced [424]. An electric potential is applied to the membrane, allowing the single-stranded DNA in the *cis*-side chamber to be electrophoretically driven through the pore [444]. At the meantime, an electric current flowing through the nanopore is also generated. As the DNA strand moves through the nanopore, the k-mer nucleotides, at the sensing region (the reader, the narrowest region) of the nanopore barrel creates a characteristic disruption to the electric current [423,445]. The current is measured by each nanopore's own electrode and utilized to determine the sequences of the polynucleotide strand, with the help of the base caller algorithms [446,447]. In addition, ONT holds the potential to identify DNA/RNA modifications such as methylation [448,449], which underlie certain diseases [450].

With these exceptional long-read sequencing technologies, both biomedical research and medicine itself have seen significant improvements. One of the most remarkable long-read sequencing accomplishments is the successful generation of the first ever complete Telomere-to-Telomere (T2T) sequence of the human genome, which introduced nearly 200 Mbp of new sequence, encompassing 1956 gene predictions, with 99 of them predicted to be protein coding [451]. T2T not only offered an improved human reference genome but also showcased the potential for long-read sequencing to make significant advancements in various aspects of genomic research, such as variant interpretation [452] and evolutionary studies [453]. Indeed, in earlier sections of this dissertation, PacBio SMRT technology was utilized to identify on- and off-target editing in the mitochondrial genome (2.4.2), while ONT sequencing was routinely employed to validate newly cloned plasmids (2.3).

4.1.2 Improving the detection and interpretation of short tandem repeats through long-read sequencing

Short tandem repeats (STRs), also known as microsatellites, are repetitive DNA sequences composed of 1- to 6-bp units. STRs comprise approximately 3% of the human genome [454], and exhibit polymorphisms and high mutation rates in the population [455]. The instability of STRs can lead to pathogenic expansions, and the underlying disease mechanism is often independent of gene function [430,456]. Several diseases, including Huntington's disease, Fragile X syndrome, and myotonic dystrophy, are associated with such regions, and the severity of these diseases is reported to correlate with the size of the repeat expansion [457]. However, accurately sequencing the repeat region presents challenges for short-read sequencing methods due to various factors. Firstly, short-read sequencing often relies on PCR-based library construction, which can undergo slippage at STR regions [458]. Secondly, the base calling of short-read sequencing machines is frequently imprecise at the STR regions [459]. Finally, pathogenic expansions can exceed the read length, making it difficult to map the reads to unique locations on the genome [460]. These limitations highlight the need for long-read sequencing technologies to address the accurate sequencing of STR regions and provide valuable insights into the understanding and diagnosis of associated diseases.

Due to the characteristics of STRs, it is hypothesized that they may potentially harbor pathogenic mutations related to numerous undiagnosed diseases [461]. For instance, utilizing the RepeatMasker data on UCSC browser, a total of 424 simple-repeat (1-6 bp) loci have been identified in 26 out of 29 genes associated with LGMD (among the genes checked, *HNRNPDL*, *TCAP*, and *GMPPB* showed no hits) [462]. 17 of these loci are longer than 100 bp (Table 4.1.2.1). Improving methods and reanalyzing such loci could potentially enhance the diagnostic yield by revealing STRs in known pathogenic loci that were previously overlooked, as well as identifying new pathogenic STRs.

Chr	T2T_start	T2T_end	CAT+Liftoff_Gene	Repeat
chr2	71489701	71489842	DYSF-201	CCCT
chr2	71588326	71588824	DYSF-201	AC
chr2	71600897	71601016	DYSF-201	TG
chr2	71675087	71675720	DYSF-201	TG
chr2	71628673	71631472	DYSF-201	GT
chr2	179041753	179041891	TTN-201	TACA
chr3	8729142	8729251	CAV3-201	CT
chr5	156884419	156884794	SGCD-201	CATATA
chr5	156963060	156963218	SGCD-201	CT
chr5	157043057	157043265	SGCD-201	TA
chr5	157073483	157073612	SGCD-201	TA
chr5	157123622	157123881	SGCD-201	AT
chr5	157142009	157142151	SGCD-201	AT
chr5	156941958	156942491	SGCD-201	AATAT
chr7	16384537	16384645	CRPPA-201	AGAA
chr13	22425665	22425814	SGCG-201	AT
chr17	51033714	51034144	SGCA-201	CA

Table 4.1.2.1 Simple-repeat loci in LGMD genes. The coordinates are based on the T2T reference genome. Base mismatches are present in certain repeat units.

Our collaborators at Illumina, Dr. Egor Dolzhenko and Dr. Michael Eberle, generated a genome-wide catalog of highly polymorphic repeats during the development of ExpansionHunter [463]. To identify the genomic locations and lengths of polymorphic repeats occurring within exonic regions, we mapped the repeats in the catalog to the GENCODE v19 transcripts. Through our analysis, we identified 1438 polymorphic repeats that overlap with the exonic regions of 1339 genes (Fig. 4.1.2.2). These Illumina polymorphic repeat regions exhibit sizes ranging from 2 bp to 150 bp (Fig. 4.1.2.3). Subsequently, we sought to determine if these exonic repeats are associated with known disease-related genes. We compared the list of exonic repeats with a Mendeliome plus incidentalome gene list (https://panelapp.agha.umccr.org/) and identified 463 repeats that overlap with 423 disease-related genes (Fig. 4.1.2.2).

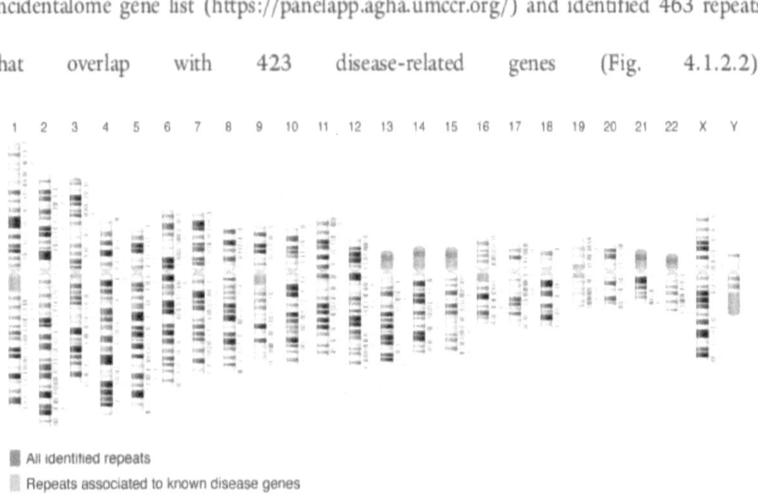

Fig. 4.1.2.2 Polymorphic repeats occurring within the exonic regions of the GENCODE v19 transcripts. Ideogram was generated using Genome Decoration Page (https://www.ncbi.nlm.nih.gov/genome/tools/gdp/).

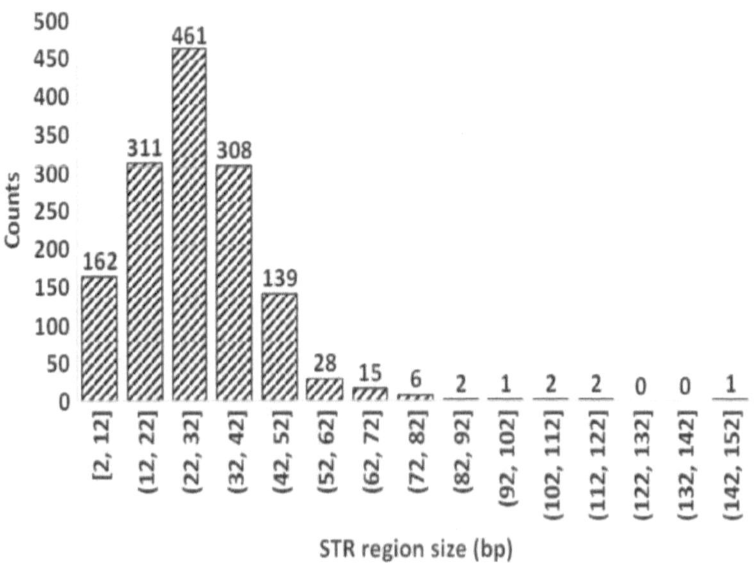

Fig. 4.1.2.3 The lengths of the polymorphic STR regions within a reference exome. The x-axis represents the sizes of the STR regions, while the y-axis represents the number of polymorphic loci falling within specific size ranges. The polymorphic loci in the human genome were identified through collaboration with Illumina. For this analysis, the exome was defined based on GENCODE annotation of "exon" and constructed using the GRCh37 reference genome data.

Although re-analysis of existing exome and genome sequencing data have potential in addressing the challenges in solving unsolved rare disease cases [464,465], it is limited by the inherent difficulties of short-read sequencing, as previously outlined. Fortunately, recent advancements in Cas9-mediated targeted capture approaches have now rendered long-read sequencing at specific genomic regions technically and economically feasible. These methods utilize Cas9 to cleave chromosomal DNA at specific loci and add adaptors at the DNA ends [466,467], enabling targeted enrichment without the need for PCR amplification. This enrichment allows for more accurate measurement of repeat copy numbers and also increases sequencing throughput.

We acquired multiple cell lines from Coriell, containing expanded STRs in different disease genes and varying STR lengths (Table 4.1.2.4). Subsequently, we cultured ~10 M cells for each line and extracted high molecular weight (HMW) genomic DNA from them using the NucleoBond HMW DNA kit (TaKaRa; 740160.20). The HMW genomic DNA of three samples (GM03621, GM07537, and GM06903) were selected and sent to the Yale Center for Genome Analysis (YCGA) for further experiments. At YCGA, the samples were examined for concentration, purity, and DNA length (Table 4.1.2.5 and Fig. 4.1.2.6). The quality of all three samples was found to be suitable for subsequent Cas9 enrichment and ONT long-read sequencing. The YCGA researchers generated long-read sequencing raw data for Sample GM03621 (expansion on *HTT*) and Sample GM06903 (expansion on *FMR1*), along with one YCGA in-house control sample each for *HTT* and *FMR1*.

ID	Description	Gene	Mutation Site
GM03561	SPINOCEREBELLAR ATAXIA 7; SCA7	ATXN7	Coding region; poly (Q)
GM06927	SPINOCEREBELLAR ATAXIA 1; SCA1	ATXN1	Coding region; poly (Q)
GM13537	SPINOCEREBELLAR ATAXIA 1; SCA1 | ATAXIN 1; ATX1	ATXN1	Coding region; poly (Q)
GM13536	SPINOCEREBELLAR ATAXIA 1; SCA1 | ATAXIN 1; ATX1	ATXN1	Coding region; poly (Q)
GM06153	MACHADO-JOSEPH DISEASE; MJD | ATAXIN 3; ATXN3	ATXN3	Coding region; poly (Q)
GM06151	MACHADO-JOSEPH DISEASE; MJD | ATAXIN 3; ATXN3	ATXN3	Coding region; poly (Q)
GM03621	HUNTINGTON DISEASE; HD	HTT	Coding region; poly (Q)
GM06903	FRAGILE X MENTAL RETARDATION SYNDROME | FMR1 GENE; FMR1	FMR1	5' UTR
GM07537	FRAGILE X MENTAL RETARDATION SYNDROME | FMR1 GENE; FMR1	FMR1	5' UTR
GM04602	DYSTROPHIA MYOTONICA 1; DM1	DMPK	Intronic

ID	Mutation type	Normal Repeat Range	Normal Allele	Expanded Allele
GM03561	(CAG)n EXPANSION	4-35	8	62
GM06927	(CAG)n EXPANSION	6-44	29	52
GM13537	(CAG)n EXPANSION	6-44	32	60
GM13536	(CAG)n EXPANSION	6-44	31	43
GM06153	(CAG)n EXPANSION	13-36	23	71
GM06151	(CAG)n EXPANSION	13-36	24	74
GM03621	(CAG)n EXPANSION	6-34	18	60
GM06903	(CGG)n EXPANSION	6-60	23	95
GM07537	(CGG)n EXPANSION	6-60	28-29	> 200
GM04602	(CTG)n EXPANSION	5-37	NA	1600-2400

Table 4.1.2.4 Coriell cell lines used for the development of long-read sequencing-based STR diagnostic methods. The data for the Normal Repeat Range were obtained from a previous review paper [457].

Sample ID	Qubit ng/uL	Nanodrop ng/uL	A260	A280	260/280	260/230	Purity
GM03621	61.5	88.2	1.765	0.947	1.86	2.34	70%
GM07537	143	108.2	2.163	1.148	1.88	2.19	76%
GM06903	83.4	102.7	2.054	1.1	1.87	2.18	81%

Table 4.1.2.5 The quality control of the HMW genomic DNA samples.

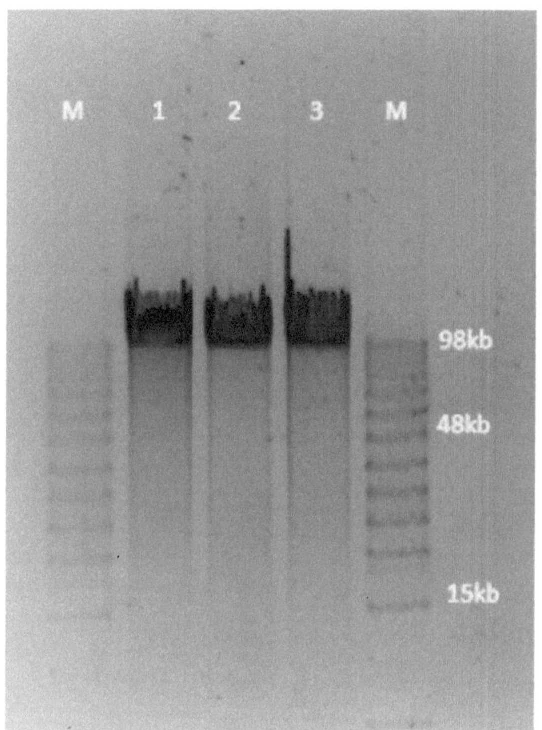

Fig. 4.1.2.6 Pulsed-field gel electrophoresis of DNA extracted from Coriell cell lines. The HMW genomic DNA from all 3 samples are in the 100-kb size range. Lane 1: GM03621, Lane 2: GM07537, Lane 3: GM06903.

Long-read sequencing reads were aligned using minimap2 to the GRCh37 reference [468], and reads surrounding the *HTT* and *FMR1* STR loci were obtained to generate the waterfall plots (Fig. 4.1.2.7). We estimated the number of repeated units using the "RepeatAnalysisTools" developed by PacBio (https://github.com/PacificBiosciences/apps-scripts/tree/master/RepeatAnalysisTools) (Table 4.1.2.8). The ONT long-read sequencing analysis accurately captured the expansion sizes of the samples, with all expected numbers falling within the 95% confidence intervals of the detected numbers.

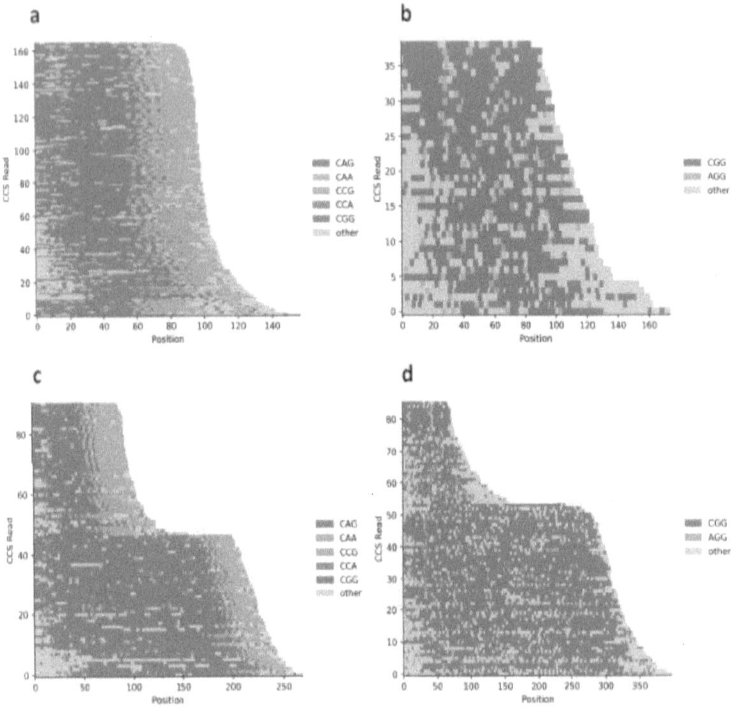

Fig. 4.1.2.7 Targeted ONT long-read sequencing of *HTT* and *FMR1* loci. The Cas9 targeted capture was performed at *HTT* and *FMR1* loci for control samples and Coriell samples. The waterfall plots illustrate each of the sequencing reads (rows) within the corresponding loci, along with the repeat length and repeat unit sequence. **a,** *HTT* control sample. **b,** *FMR1* control sample. **c,** Sample GM03621 (expansion in *HTT*). **d,** Sample GM06903 (expansion in *FMR1*).

Samples	Range in healthy individuals	Expected allele 1	Detected allele 1	Expected allele 2	Detected allele 2
HTT control	6-34	\	13.9 (8-17)	\	19 (16-22)
FMR1 control	6-60	\	25.5 (18-29)	\	21 (18-25)
GM03621 (*HTT*)	6-34	18	16 (10-20)	60	51 (37-60)
GM06903 (*FMR1*)	6-60	23	20 (12-24)	95	83.5 (53-95)

Table 4.1.2.8 The repeat sizes determined by long-read sequencing at the *HTT* and *FMR1* loci. The numbers in the parentheses indicate the 95% confidence intervals. The expected allele sizes are unknown for the control samples as no other approaches has been used to determine them. The data for the Normal Repeat Range were obtained from a previous review paper [457].

To further increase the throughput of long-read sequencing at targeted STR loci, one approach is to design and optimize Cas9 sgRNAs to simultaneously target multiple STR loci of interest. Notably, it has been reported that four regions can be captured simultaneously [469]. By modifying the experimental procedures and analytical pipelines, the throughput may be further enhanced. Additionally, utilizing barcoding strategies can enable the simultaneous sequencing of samples from multiple individuals, further improving the capability of Cas9-mediated targeted capture approaches [470].

Finally, the continuous efforts to lower the costs linked with long-read sequencing are progressively opening avenues for the eventual shift towards whole-genome sequencing on a broader population scale [471,472]. Considering the notable variability of STR sites, the creation of a comprehensive population reference panel becomes crucial for distinguishing between normal and potentially pathogenic variations. The advent of more cost-effective long-read sequencing is expected to facilitate the establishment of such a panel, enabling enhanced accuracy in STR variant interpretation.

4.2 Future assays towards a comprehensive Variant Effects Atlas

4.2.1 Overview of functional assays compatible with DMS

A comprehensive Variant Effects Atlas has the potential to revolutionize diagnostics, but there is still a long way to go. Fortunately, the availability of numerous assays specifically designed for studying various disease mechanisms provides a valuable opportunity for their adaptation to DMS applications. This section of the dissertation serves as a prospect to introduce a variety of functional assays that can be used in a high-throughput manner or have the potential to be adapted for high-throughput use in different broad disease mechanisms. A specific focus is placed on cost-effective methods that do not require robotics or automation. Instead, these methods employ well-designed molecular tools to transform biological mechanisms into easily detectable signals, such as fluorescence, drug resistance, or cell survival rates.

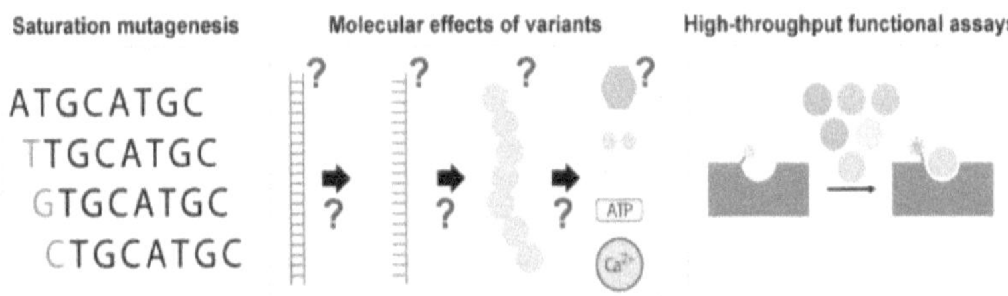

Fig. 4.2.1.1 Selection of functional assays for DMS. Functional assays suitable for DMS should bridge molecular effects of variants to detectable signals, like fluorescence markers or growth enrichment. These assays are preferred to have high-throughput capabilities to handle pooled samples resulting from saturation mutagenesis. Molecular effects to be detected encompass DNA replication, repair, or modification; RNA transcription, maturation, transport, or stability; protein abundance or misfolding; protein modification or localization; and various metabolites such as sugars, lipids, ATP, and ions.

Prior to discussing various disease mechanisms and their corresponding functional assays, it's important to highlight the bioreceptor-based assays. Bioreceptors are biological or biomimetic components that recognize the target analyte and produce measurable signals that are proportional to the concentration of the analyte. The most widely used bioreceptors are antibodies. Originating from the immune system, antibodies possess remarkable versatilities, allowing them to specifically bind various antigens, which include not only proteins but also DNAs [473], RNAs [474], lipids [475] and sugars [476]. Haptens are small molecules with sizes smaller than 1 kDa, *e.g.*, neurotransmitters including serotonin and dopamine [477]. They can be recognized by corresponding antibodies when attached to larger protein carriers, like albumins, thyroglobulins, hemocyanins and polylysine [478].

In addition to traditional antibodies, newly developed bioreceptors offer simplified designs and manufacturing processes [479]. Fragment antibodies, like scFv [480], contain only the functional regions of antibodies, which increase their specificity and penetrability. Aptamers, including oligonucleotides [481] and short peptides [482], can be programmatically designed and manufactured to selectively bind to specific targets. This design flexibility arises from their standardized composition, such as the four nucleotides in DNA aptamers. Consequently, aptamers can undergo directed evolution, enabling the rapid generation of new aptamers tailored to specific targets. The most commonly used method for selecting specific aptamers is the Systematic Evolution of Ligands by EXponential Enrichment (SELEX), which involves screening a library of random sequences to identify aptamers for a desired target [483]. Other small-molecule tools include ligand-dependent transcription factors and riboswitch, and FRET systems that generate a fluorescence signal when two molecules bind together [484].

Given the generalizability of bioreceptor-based assays, it is advisable to begin DMS functional assay design by searching for existing bioreceptors or creating new ones before considering alternative assays.

On the other hand, while DMS holds promising potential, it is crucial to consider certain limitations associated with its application. Many available functional assays were originally developed for purposes other than variant interpretation, such as gene discoveries which required lower sensitivity of assays. Further optimization for these assays might be needed to improve the sensitivity and dynamic range.

Another caveat of the DMS workflows is that both the experimental design and the data analysis are dependent on one assumption that the disease mechanism in question is exclusively responsible for the symptoms. However, this assumption is not always true, as many genes have multiple functions and different variants of these genes may lead to distinctly unrelated diseases through different pathological pathways [485].

Additionally, in certain scenarios, a variant can have an impact on multiple levels of molecular processes. For example, if the variants of interest are located within the coding sequence, the disease mechanisms may involve effects on both the RNA level and the protein level. Therefore, it may be necessary to explore and assess these effects on both levels with relevant assays.

It is important to bear in mind that the DMS is often only capable of investigating one aspect of the gene functions. Hence, it may conceal the pathogenicity of some variants and lead to inaccurate classification of these variants. For instance, sarcoglycanopathies are a group of diseases caused by genetic defects in four cell membrane glycoproteins, α-, β-, γ- and δ-sarcoglycan. These four sarcoglycans form a complex at muscle cell membrane to carry out their function [486]. The abundance, conformation, assembly and localization of the sarcoglycans may have cross-interaction effects, making it hard to evaluate all variants with a single DMS assay. To address this issue, orthogonal assays evaluating different factors should be considered and added into the DMS workflow.

4.2.2 Assays for diseases related to DNA replication, repair, or modification

DNA is the fundamental bearer of genetic information. Essentially, all genetic diseases are due to DNA changes. This session primarily emphasizes disease mechanisms that disrupt the biochemical properties of DNA rather than its sequence. DNA replication and repair are essential for development and homeostasis [487], malfunctions of which can lead to birth defects, *e.g.*, Meier-Gorlin syndrome [488] and accelerated aging disorders [489]. DNA modifications are essential for expression regulation, transposon silencing, and DNA repairing [490], and are associated with imprinting disorders [491]. The variants leading to DNA disturbances can be either via *in situ* effects specific to the mutational sequence that alters the DNA modifications or DNA replication origin motifs, or by deactivating complex machinery involved in repair systems.

Due to the essential role of maintaining DNA integrity, gene mutations in these associated pathways are likely to have consequences impacting cell viability. Therefore, cell growth enrichments are simple high-throughput assays for evaluating variants, where those that negatively impact cell viability and/or proliferation are gradually eliminated, resulting in an enrichment of variants that have neutral functional impact. DMS has been used to study the impact genetic mutations have on DNA mismatch repair (MMR), which involves the detection and repair of erroneous sequences on the newly synthesized DNA strand that arise during DNA replication, recombination or the repair of DNA damage [492]. *MSH2* is a gene involved in MMR, where loss-of-function variants are associated with Lynch syndrome, conferring predisposition to cancers, particularly colorectal cancers. A recent study in *MSH2* elegantly utilized the purine analog, 6-

thioguanine (6-TG), which triggers MMR and leads to cell death when incorporated into DNA. Thus, *MSH2* loss-of-function variants that have defective MMR are resistant to the toxic effects of 6-TG and cell growth enrichment assay can be utilized to select these damaging variants [184]. This assay can be adapted for other MMR-related genes including *MSH6* [493] and *MLH1* [494]. Additionally, to enhance the lethality and strength of selection in these growth enrichment assays, a commonly employed approach is to introduce genetic predisposition by introducing mutations in related genes in model cell lines prior to performing the assay. For instance, the knockout of *PARP14* was performed to identify essential genes for the viability of PARP14-deficient cells [495].

DNA replication and damage can also be directly detected using a fluorescent reporter. The nucleoside analogues Bromodeoxyuridine (BrdU) and 5-Ethynyl-2'-deoxyuridine (EdU) are commonly used to quantify DNA replication, where they are incorporated into nascent DNA, generating detectable signals. The detection of BrdU is antibody-based and can quantify DNA damage by labeling the double-strand breaks [496]. In contrast, the detection of EdU utilizes "click chemistry" to conjugate fluorochrome-tagged azides with EdUs [497]. Incorporated EdU can be removed by the nucleotide excision repair (NER) [498]. Hence, EdU-based assays also have the potential to assist variant interpretation for diseases associated with the NER pathway. Mutations in the NER pathway are associated with xeroderma pigmentosum (XP) that causes severe sunburn and Cockayne syndrome (CS), a developmental disorder that results in severely reduced lifespans [499]. The nine genes currently associated with XP and two genes linked to CS can be further studied employing these fluorescent reporter assays. Flow cytometry-based nucleoside analogue assays have been developed and utilized to evaluate cell proliferation in type-1 diabetes and norepinephrine depleted hippocampal cells [500] or evaluate DNA damage responses triggered by either UV or DNA topoisomerase I inhibitor topotecan (Tpt) [501]. Such assays opened the door to high-throughput variant interpretation.

Various alternative strategies have emerged for cytometric detection of DNA damage either by utilizing nucleic acid binding dyes like acridine orange [502] or by targeting the factors recruited to the breakpoints [503,504]. Additional methods to evaluate DNA damage include high-throughput microscopy [505] and array-based assays [506].

4.2.3 Assays for diseases related to RNA transcription, maturation, transport, or stability

RNA, specifically mRNA, serves as a connecting agent between the genetic information encoded in DNA and the biological function executed by protein. As a result, RNA regulation is crucial to the correct pattern and level of gene expression [507].

To evaluate variants associated with transcriptional misregulation disorders [508], a universal strategy for characterizing transcription regulation in a high-throughput manner is through using the reporter assays via endogenous knock-in [80,509] or exogenous reporter constructs. The endogenous knock-in reserves the correct genomic context and hence may better reveal the *in vivo* regulation landscape. Assays employing exogenous reporter constructs lose the genomic context but can be easily performed on a larger scale for regulatory elements of multiple genes. One frequently used assay that utilizes exogenous reporter constructs is Massively Parallel Reporter Assay (MPRA) [510], where variants are introduced to their respective constructs and characterized according to the reporter signals in parallel [511,512]. In the study performed by Melnikov et al., each construct contained an enhancer that carried either a single-hit variant or multi-hit variants, an invariant promoter, a *luc2* luciferase gene and a unique sequencing tag that is used to identify the variant(s) in this construct. Genome-wide association studies (GWAS) identified numerous schizophrenia (SZ) and Alzheimer's disease (AD) associated variants that were hypothesized to affect gene transcription. An MPRA study was performed to evaluate these variants [513], where each construct carried a GWAS-associated variant, a minimal promoter, a green fluorescent protein (GFP) and a sequencing tag. In both aforementioned studies, the variant effects on gene expression were assessed through the enrichment of sequencing tags rather than the signal strength of the luciferase/GFP. This approach was adopted because a single cell could contain multiple constructs, and the reporter signal did not straightforwardly reflect the enhancer activity. Site-specific integration provides additional enhancements to MPRA, where each cell is controlled to carry only one construct. This method was developed in an MPRA for identification of mammalian enhancers [514], where each construct in the pool contained a sheared genomic sequence (~1-1.6 kb) that was being evaluated for enhancer activity, a minimal promoter and a yellow fluorescent protein (YFP), whose signal was used to quantify the enhancer activity. This strategy made it possible to perform MPRA using an FFC assay.

Post-transcriptional regulations modulate RNA splicing and RNA stability. These mechanisms are closely linked to spliceosomopathies [515] and RNA degradation disorders

[516]. MPRA-based methods can be adapted to examine post-transcriptional regulations. To specifically study splicing, the variants can be included in an artificial region inserted either in a canonical exon or a canonical intron. Different splicing events in this region may switch on/off one reporter, *e.g.*, Multiplexed Functional Assay of Splicing using Sort-seq (MFASS) [517], or two reporters in different frames [518]. MPRA-based assays can also be utilized to assess the potential functional effects of variants located in the 5'UTR and 3'UTR on transcript levels. For instance, Pooled full-length UTR Multiplex Assay on Gene Expression (PLUMAGE) was employed to identify functional 5'UTR SNVs in prostate cancer [519]. MPRA for 3'UTRs (MPRAu) identified a variant that regulates the viral defense gene *TRIM14* and another variant that modifies *PILRB* abundance, nominating a causal variant in age-related macular degeneration [520].

Proper RNA function also relies on its localization. MPRA-based methods can be modified to quantify subcellular compartmental enrichment, enabling their application in the study of diseases related to RNA mislocalization. For instance, annexin, encoded by *ANXA11*, connects RNA granules to lysosomal membranes. Mutations in *ANXA11* perturb the transport system that delivers RNA to distal parts of neurites. This disruption leads to amyotrophic lateral sclerosis (ALS), a disease characterized by reduced muscle functionality and nerve cell breakdown [521]. In neurons, RNA from soma and neurite compartments can be collected separately, allowing identification of variants that affect RNA transport [522]. Nuclear-retained long non-coding RNAs (lncRNAs) can serve as key regulators of gene expression. A notable example is MALAT1, one of the most abundant nuclear-retained lncRNAs, which facilitates transcriptional activation and is associated with cancer metastasis [523]. Massively Parallel RNA Assay (MPRNA) can evaluate the nuclear enrichment of RNA by isolating the nuclei from the cells, which identified unique nuclear localization domains of nuclear lncRNAs [524]. Both aforementioned assays require separate collection of different subcellular compartments, which may be sophisticated to perform. APEX-seq is a proximity labeling technique, which can be utilized to isolate RNAs from various subcellular compartments [525]. APEX-seq utilizes the peroxidase enzyme APEX2 that is genetically targeted to the cellular region of interest to biotinylate RNA molecules within a few nanometers of APEX2. Such biotinylated RNA can be isolated using streptavidin-coated beads. APEX-seq holds promise as a universal assay for RNA localization independent from separate collection of different compartments.

4.2.4 Assays for diseases related to protein abundance or misfolding

(Kaiyue Ma and Shushu Huang)

Proteins are the chief actors of cellular functions. Damaging missense variants are often a result of amino acid substitutions with significantly different biochemical properties that have two broad effects on protein structure and abundance. Firstly, missense variants can contribute to decreased translation efficiency or stability associated with translation deregulation disorders [526]. In addition, missense variants can lead to misfolding resulting in proteinopathies [527] which comprise a large variety of diseases, notably cystic fibrosis [528] and Alzheimer's disease [529]. Lastly, the overall reduction of protein levels underlies the majority of haploinsufficient diseases.

Variant Abundance by Massively Parallel Sequencing (VAMP-seq) [530] is a universal assay that screens variants affecting protein abundance. VAMP-seq utilizes a plasmid pool of variants in a gene of interest fused to eGFP that is then integrated into cells through recombination. Variants impacting the abundance of the target protein should result in a lower fluorescent signal. Applying VAMP-seq, Matreyek et al. evaluated the single amino acid variants of *PTEN*, a tumor suppressor gene, and showed selection for low abundance *PTEN* variants as a common oncogenic mechanism. They also screened variants in *TPMT*, which encodes thiopurine methyltransferase whose activity is associated with the toxicity of thiopurine drugs widely used in the treatment of acute lymphoblastic leukemia (ALL). Furthermore, it has been inferred that employing C-term tagged eGFP in addition to regular VAMP-seq may allow the assessment of variant effects on protein conformation [531]. The main limitation of VAMP-seq is its reliance on eGFP that can be overcome using small-sized epitope tags (*e.g.*, FLAG) accompanied with their corresponding antibodies. The general VAMP-seq framework is a simple yet powerful tool that empowers the study of a broad range of disease mechanisms, where sufficient protein abundance is required for normal function.

Secreted proteins play crucial roles in mediating communication between cells, and perturbations in the secretome are implicated in the pathogenesis of metabolic disorders, cancer, and neurodegenerative diseases. [532]. However, since secreted proteins function outside the cell membrane, they become disassociated from the cells that produced them. Consequently, this makes them unsuitable for DMS assays like VAMP-seq, which rely on isolating cellular DNA that produces the corresponding mutant protein [533]. Gel Microdroplet-Fluorescence Activated Cell Sorting (GMD-FACS) can address this issue by encapsulating single cells and their secreted proteins in gel microdroplets (GMDs) [534]. Fang et al. employed GMD-FACS to link individual yeast cells with the monoclonal antibodies (mAbs) they secreted. This demonstrates that this assay can be adapted to assess variant impact on the corresponding secreted protein levels.

The malfunction of certain proteins may not be evident in isolation, as they rely on interactions with other molecules. Examples can be observed in cell-to-cell interactions in the central nervous system which play crucial roles in neurological diseases [535,536]. Systematic perturbation of encapsulated associated cells followed by sequencing (SPEAC-seq) was developed as a droplet-based high-throughput platform that enables forward genetic screens of cell-cell interaction mechanisms [537]. This assay involved the co-encapsulation and co-culturing of two cells within droplets, allowing them to remain isolated from neighboring cell pairs. These cells interacted through direct contact and/or the exchange of secreted soluble factors. Upon successful interaction between these two cells, the cell pair exhibits reporter activation, *e.g.*, EGFP, which can be detected and captured through droplet sorting. SPEAC-seq has the potential to evaluate variants in genes that are involved in cell-to-cell interaction.

4.2.5 Assays for diseases related to protein modification or localization

de novo Protein expression from DNA sequence is energetically expensive and imposes a time delay in generating a response. In contrast, post-translational modifications and translocalization of existing proteins enable rapid and efficient responses to cellular changes. Mutations affecting these processes can contribute to various diseases [538].

Variants that impact acetylation, glycosylation, methylation and other protein modifications can cause various types of diseases [539]. An example is a group of diseases termed dystroglycanopathies, which result from hypoglycosylation of alpha-dystroglycan (alpha-DG) [146]. For DMS studies focusing on post-translational modifications (PTMs), methods relying on bioreceptors are prioritized choices due to their compatibility with pooled saturation mutagenesis. For example, IIH6C4 is an antibody specific to glycosylated alpha-DG, and can be coupled to flow cytometry [177]. This cytometric assay was developed to evaluate the alpha-DG glycosylation in patient fibroblasts with mutations in associated enzymes, but can be easily adapted for DMS studies to improve functional variant interpretation for more than a dozen of enzymes involved in alpha-DG glycosylation. In addition, nanopore technologies provide an alternative and more generalizable method for detection of PTMs [540], which utilize ionic current signals to identify different PTMs. This potentially can be developed into high-throughput assays [541] by fusing the target proteins with unique barcode peptides. Nanopore can identify the PTMs on the target proteins as well as the fused barcode peptides, which can be linked to specific consequences.

Proper functioning of many proteins relies on their designated compartments, which are often specified by their signal peptides [542]. Protein mislocalization acts as a disease mechanism, leading to protein inactivation or toxic misregulation. An interesting example is observed in primary hyperoxaluria type 1 (PH1), where the enzyme AGT is mislocalized from peroxisomes to the mitochondria [543]. Mislocalizations can be studied using assays such as HiLITR (High-throughput Localization Indicator with

Transcriptional Readout) that converts protein localization information into detectable fluorescent signals [544]. In HiLITR, a TEV protease is programmed to localize at a given site, for instance, the mitochondrial surface or the endoplasmic reticulum (ER) surface, and a transcription factor (TF) is fused to the protein-of-interest (POI) via a linker containing a TEV cutting site (TEVcs). Upon colocalization of the POI and the TEV, the TF is released and can subsequently turn on the expression of a fluorescence protein regulated by this TF. By applying HiLITR, Coukos et al. discovered that *SAE1* and *EMC10* were associated with mislocalization of mitochondrial and ER proteins. HiLITR has the potential to be adapted for other subcellular localizations. For instance, instead of being fused to TEVcs-TF, the POI can be fused to dark-to-bright protease reporters carrying TEVcs, like FlipGFP [545] or cyclic mNeonGreen2 [546]. By adding a mitochondrial targeting sequence (MTS) to both the TEV protease and the POI-reporter fusion protein, the variant effects on mitochondrial localization can be evaluated. In addition, high-throughput microscopy enhanced with deep learning can be employed to identify specific subcellular compartments and assess protein localization. A study demonstrated an example where the authors successfully achieved accurate classification of protein localization for 12 subcellular compartments [547].

4.2.6 Assays for diseases related to different metabolites

Many metabolites impact cell viability by interfering with nutrient biosynthesis and utilization or by accumulating toxicity, which lead to inherited metabolic disorders, encompassing a wide range of diseases [548].

Growth assays can be developed for variants associated with these metabolites. A commonly used strategy utilizes yeast surrogate platforms, where the yeast orthologous gene is deleted and replaced with the human ortholog carrying the variant of interest. In a recent study, the functional effects of SNV-accessible single amino acid substitutions were assessed in the human *OTC* gene, which encodes ornithine transcarbamylase (OTC) and is linked to the most prevalent urea cycle disorder [549]. In this study, the human *OTC* was incorporated into a yeast strain lacking the yeast ortholog *ARG3* gene. As *ARG3/OTC* is required for yeast to grow on arginine-deficient medium, *OTC* variants that are depleted from the arginine-deficient growth assay can be identified as likely pathogenic variants.

Methods relying on bioreceptors are alternative preferred choices. Below are three example assays with relatively broad applicability. ATP is the primary energy carrier in cells and a universal substrate of kinases. This makes ATP level a generalized functional reflection of the kinase activities. In a flow cytometry-based assay for ATP [550], a FRET system was employed to generate ATP-dependent signals, which consisted of a modified cyan fluorescent protein (CFP) and a monomeric Venus (mVenus) separated by an ATP-binding domain. With this assay, the authors identified ATP-critical genes, revealing an enrichment in mitochondrial pathways. Interestingly, the authors also identified ATP-critical genes not known to be involved in energy metabolism, namely *SLC30A9* and *SNRPD3*. Besides ATP, another important metabolite in energy metabolism is glucose, which serves as the primary energy source. There has also been a FRET flow cytometry developed for glucose, which utilizes a FRET pair consisting of an enhanced cyan fluorescent protein (ECFP) and an mCitrine separated by a glucose binding domain [551].

The last example is an assay specifically designed for lipid droplets (LDs), which are crucial in energy supply and cellular homeostasis. A fluorescent biosensor called C-Py was designed and synthesized to specifically target the LDs, which is compatible with flow cytometry [552].

In addition, assays that rely on microtiter plates are available for different metabolites, like fluorometric assays for ATP [553]. Assays for lipids include colorimetric assays [554] and fluorometric assays based on either fluorescence quenching [555] or FRET [556]. Assays for sugars include colorimetric assays [557] and near-infrared spectroscopy (NIRS) [558]. A notable example is the enzyme cascade fluorescence-based assay [559] for the quantification of phenylalanine, which is accumulated to toxic levels in Phenylketonuria (PKU) due to phenylalanine hydroxylase mutations [560]. The scale of these assays can be significantly increased by incorporating microdroplet approaches, enabling massively parallel reactions to occur within individual microdroplets [561].

4.2.7 Assays for diseases related to ions

(Frances Cheung and Kaiyue Ma)

Cells actively regulate ion concentrations and establish electric membrane potentials to support vital physiological processes, including development, regeneration, cell communication, and other essential activities. For instance, mitochondria rely on ion gradients to generate energy, while organs like the heart, brain, and skeletal muscles function through action potentials [562]. Disruptions to these processes can give rise to conditions like arrhythmia, cardiomyopathy, epilepsy, Parkinson's disease, chronic pain, and autoimmune disorders such as multiple sclerosis [563].

Recently, DMS via adapting a three-drug cytotoxicity assay was able to discern wild-type from gain- and loss-of-function pathogenic variants in a library of nearly all possible *SCN5A* variants [564]. *SCN5A* encodes a major voltage-gated sodium cardiac channel, whose mutations can lead to genetic arrhythmias, atrial fibrillations, dilated cardiomyopathies, and other heart conditions. The cytotoxicity assay utilized 2 sodium channel agonists, veratridine and brevetoxin, and an $Na+/K+$ exchange inhibitor, ouabain. The sodium channel agonists result in open state sodium channels, which lead to sodium influx, and the ouabain results in increased sensitivity to sodium overload. As a result, cells expressing functional sodium channels undergo cell death. When variants are treated with this triple-drug mixture, there is a graded response for cell survival, with gain-of-function mutations having decreased viability and loss-of-function mutations having increased viability.

Ion channels are becoming attractive drug targets for an increasing number of disease indications. For instance, zinc is an essential protein structural constituent for receptors, enzymes, transcription factors, growth factors, and others, and about 10% of all proteins bind zinc. The biological functions of these proteins are dependent on cellular zinc levels, and deficiencies in zinc binding can lead to immunodeficiencies, growth retardation, cancer progressions, and other health problems [565].

Ion fluorescent indicators can be utilized for studying ion homeostasis and potentially developing high-throughput screening assays. They are categorized into three types: small-molecule, genetically encoded, or hybrid [566]. Sensors in all classes consist of a metal-binding group and at least one fluorophore. Small-molecule probes are exogenous compounds that are either intensity-based, meaning they increase fluorescence intensity, or ratiometric, meaning they shift excitation and/or emission wavelengths. Genetically encoded sensors are fluorescent proteins attached to ion binding proteins, such as Zn^{2+} binding proteins. Currently, most genetically encoded Zn^{2+} sensors are FRET-based and monitor Zn^{2+} levels via FRET efficiency. While FRET-based sensors are preferred for quantifications, single fluorescent protein-based sensors have recently been popular for their ability to be multiplexed with other fluorescent sensors and for their greater dynamic ranges [567]. Such sensors have more commonly been developed for Ca^{2+}, and have recently been optimized for high-throughput screening of Ca^{2+} channels. For instance, Wu et al. coupled the indicator GCaMP6 with a blasticidin selection marker via a self-cleaving peptide, allowing them to create stable-expressing 293-F clonal cell lines for intracellular calcium assays. Similar Zn^{2+} sensors are in the process of being engineered [568]. Finally, hybrid probes have both genetically encoded and exogenous components. Two such systems that have been developed are the SNAP-tag system that targets specific cellular locations [569] and the carbonic anhydrase platform that is capable of being used for imaging tissues.

Fluorescent bioelectricity reporters (FBRs) have gained significant popularity as a viable option in studying electrophysiological characteristics [562]. FBRs are fluorescent dyes that are categorized based on the response speed to membrane potential changes. Slow-response probes function by physically moving in and out of the cell or between the lipid bilayer leaflets. These probes are generally lipophilic cations or anions that translocate across membranes via electrophoretic mechanisms, and change fluorescence based on potential-dependent changes in transmembrane distribution. They are typically used to measure biological activities that occur over long timescales, such as slow metabolic processes [570]. Fast-response probes respond to changes by undergoing conformational changes, which occur quicker than the physical movement of slow-response probes. Specifically, when there is a change to the electric field, the probes undergo an intramolecular change in electronic structure and ultimately fluorescence properties. These are usually more optimal for studying rapid changes in bioelectricity, such as action potentials. FBRs hold potential for being adapted to high-throughput microscopy applications.

4.3 Searching for muscle repair solutions in biodiversity

A crucial domain of biomedicine research lies in discovering innovative therapeutic avenues that can offer safer, more economical, and highly efficient treatments, ultimately contributing to the advancement of healthcare. Evolution can be considered as the largest trial-and-error experiment in biology by far, and biodiversity presents a tremendous opportunity to discover remarkable biomedical tools. Notably, two of the most revolutionary biomedical tools, PCR and CRISPR, were both derived from discoveries in biodiversity [571,572]. Scientists devoted to the conservation and exploration of biodiversity share a collective vision that biodiversity harbors valuable genetic resources and promising healthcare opportunities [573].

With gene therapy, it is feasible to halt further muscle disease deterioration. However, treatments capable of repairing existing damage, particularly those that can complement gene therapy designed for genetic muscle diseases, still require further in-depth investigation. This section of the dissertation delves into the future prospects of exploring muscle repair solutions in biodiversity.

Muscle or muscle-like tissues are found across Planulozoa, a diverse taxonomic clade comprising species ranging from corals to mammals. Many of these species possess unique traits, including muscle regeneration and resistance to muscle damage, and could lead to therapeutic opportunities [574].

In the context of muscle diseases, muscle damages frequently occur during physical exertion. Fast-moving species, such as cheetahs, are believed to have mechanisms that can mitigate muscle damage [575]. Deep-sea species also possess unique muscle traits, contributing to their ability of withstanding high pressures. These traits include enzymatic activities [576] and unique protein stabilizers such as trimethylamine oxide (TMAO), a metabolite important for the deep-sea inhabitation [577]. Therapeutic opportunities that can strengthen muscle resistance to damage may reside in these species.

For instance, extracellular matrix (ECM) is highly involved in resistance to muscle damage [578], and a mammalian embryonic ECM protein, Laminin 111, has demonstrated therapeutic efficacy in enhancing muscle strength, resistance and post-damage muscle repair [579].

In addition, the mammalian-conserved microRNA miR-486 has shown beneficial effects on reducing muscle pathology [580]. A noteworthy observation is that miR-486 was found to be truncated in gibbons, a member of the Hominoidea (apes) taxonomic group (Fig. 4.3.1), which makes gibbons an even more interesting primate model to study muscle-related physiology [581]. Another interesting observation is that miR-486 is missing in marsupials, including opossums, Tasmanian devils, and wallabies (Fig. 4.3.1). While the specific relevance of this absence is currently unknown, it is worth noting that many marsupials are known to be susceptible to capture myopathy, a condition that can occur in animals subjected to stress during capture and handling [582-585]. Further research on miR-486 and its role in marsupials may provide valuable insights into muscle-related physiology and potential links to conditions like capture myopathy in these species. However, it must be noted that these genomic observations might have been influenced by sequencing or assembly errors. Further validations are needed before diving into any research.

Muscle regeneration in lower vertebrates, such as fish and amphibians, can be remarkable [586]. For example, zebrafish can regenerate heart muscles by mobilizing existing cardiomyocytes [587]. In contrast, injured human hearts fail to regenerate and can lead to heart failure. Lower vertebrates offer potential for identifying genomic mechanisms underlying cellular mobilization that may be partly conserved in humans and can be enhanced as a therapy for repairing damaged muscle.

Fig. 4.3.1 miR-486 is highly conserved in mammals. Light blue highlights an inverted duplicated element with the following sequence: TCCTGTACTGAGCTGCCCCGAG.

There are two main approaches for comparative genomics studies: (1) identifying genomic regions that are evolving at a faster rate than neutral evolution in certain species groups, and (2) identifying regions that are conserved among species sharing a particular trait. Both approaches contribute to a better understanding of the relationship between the genome and traits in biodiversity.

An example for Approach1 is the study of human accelerated regions (HARs) [588]. HARs are genomic regions that are conserved through evolution but significantly different in humans, presumably correlating with intelligence. Computational tools such as substitution models and likelihood ratio tests have been established in previous HARs studies to identify genomic variations. These tools can be adapted to study muscle-related traits, comparing the species of interest with their related species that lack the trait of interest. Genomic sequences of these species are available in databases like Genome10k [589].

An example for Approach2 is the Zoonomia project, which identified genetic constraints in 240 mammalian species [590]. While the Zoonomia project did not focus on muscle traits, it provided valuable tools that can be adapted for the muscle-related research. The Zoonomia tools were applied to qualitative traits like hibernation and vocal learning, as well as quantitative traits like brain size. These applications open up possibilities for utilizing these tools in studying muscle-related qualitative and quantitative traits, such as presence/absence of cellular mobilization and maximum stress capacity of muscle fibers. These tools include: [1] The "Cactus" aligner, designed to align a massive number of genomes in the thousand-genome era. [2] The constraint scoring method, developed to identify the conservation of single DNA bases across numerous species. [3] Tools like RERconverge, developed to associate specific traits with genomic sequences of different species.

In addition to comparative genomics studies, a comprehensive search for metabolites/compounds that can modulate the muscle function-related metabolic pathways can further accelerate identification of therapeutic opportunities in biodiversity. This requires using pathway database mining tools like KEGG mapper and deep-learning algorithms like DeepRF to associate metabolites/genes with the pathways they participate in and identify potential drug candidates[591,592].

The pathway search should be expanded beyond Planulozoa, as the metabolites of interest may also exist in other biological kingdoms, including microorganisms and medicinal plants. Since the metabolites can be linked to diverse pathways in different organisms, they present both therapeutic opportunities and potential risks for translational applications. For example, TMAO can increase muscle contractility, potentially through human cardiometabolic pathways [593], but is also associated with gut microbiota-related inflammation [594]. A comprehensive cross-kingdom search can improve our understanding of the benefits and risks.

Pathway searching has shown potential in a drug discovery project for FSHD within my PhD lab. Mitochondrial oxidative stress-related pathways are crucial in FSHD pathology [595]. Interestingly, Honokiol, a compound derived from magnolia trees, has also been reported to modulate these pathways likely as a defense mechanism against pests/pathogens [596,597]. Honokiol showed therapeutic efficacy in FSHD disease model cell line [598]. Additionally, FKRP catalyzes the extension of alpha-dystroglycan sugar chain with RboP, a metabolite that is only recently identified in mammals but a major component of the cell wall in Gram-positive bacteria [599]. Drug candidates that regulate RboP transfer may be identified in these bacteria. Similarly, pathway search can facilitate the identification of drug candidates for other muscle disease-related pathways.

Muscle therapeutic opportunities abound in biodiversity. As I chart my future research plan, my aim is to explore this vast resource and uncover novel discoveries that can be translated into practical applications [600,601].

Concluding Remarks

Original contributions and advancement to the field:

This thesis is dedicated to two crucial dimensions aimed at accelerating the quest for cures in the realm of rare muscle diseases: the enhancement of diagnostics and the development of innovative pathways in treatment development.

This dissertation lays the foundation for a deep mutational scanning framework known as Saturation Mutagenesis-Reinforced Functional assays (SMuRF). SMuRF is designed to be adaptable, simple, and cost-effective, with the aim of enhancing variant interpretation. SMuRF's utility was validated through its application to dystroglycanopathies, a group of rare muscle diseases arising from mutations in enzymes linked to alpha-dystroglycan glycosylation, including FKRP and LARGE1.

The SMuRF screen assessed over 99.9% of all possible coding single nucleotide variants (SNVs) in *FKRP* and *LARGE1*. It enhanced variant classification, provided training datasets for computational predictors, and elucidated critical enzyme regions for diverse disease mechanisms. SMuRF was developed to enhance accessibility for research laboratories within the rare disease field, presenting a simple and economical approach in a context where previously available methods proved either prohibitively expensive or excessively complex to implement, thus constituting an original contribution to the rare disease research community.

Additionally, the thesis provides an in-depth and comprehensive narrative detailing the intricacies of an individualized gene therapy development process for a Duchenne muscular dystrophy patient with dystrophin muscle isoform exon1 deletion. A strategy called Substitute Isoform Rescue (SIR) was employed for this gene therapy, which harnessed the redundancy within genomes for therapeutic purposes. Specifically, the SIR strategy entailed the up-regulation of the cortical isoform of dystrophin, an almost identical substitute for the muscle isoform, using a CRISPR-activation (CRISPRa) construct. The efficacy of this therapeutic strategy was demonstrated through a series of pre-clinical experiments conducted in human model cell lines, patient-specific cell lines, and an hDMD/mdx2 mouse model. Notably, the U.S. Food and Drug Administration (FDA) issued a "Safe to Proceed" letter for the Investigational New Drug (IND) application aimed at delivering the construct via AAV9, paving the way for an n-of-1 clinical trial (NCT05514249) at UMass Medical School (UMMS).

The therapeutic strategy utilized in the clinical trial highlights SIR as a viable approach to leverage genomic redundancy for genetic rescue, opening up a new avenue of exploration in gene therapy. Additionally, this development process exemplifies a gene therapy trajectory capable of rapid advancement, operating independently of large pharmaceutical companies. It also underscores critical efficacy and safety considerations, especially pertinent for older patients exhibiting advanced symptoms. These insights offer potential benefits to the broader rare disease community, constituting a modest yet previously absent addition to the existing knowledge in the field.

www.ingramcontent.com/pod-product-compliance
Lightning Source LLC
LaVergne TN
LVHW091307150826
845673LV00006B/1572

* 9 7 8 3 3 8 4 3 4 3 2 5 3 *